Contents

KU-156-187

		Page
■	Why Do We Need to Assess Competence? *Sir Rex Richards*	6
■	Clinical Performance in the National Health Service, *Liam Donaldson*	17
■	The Principles and Practice of Assessing Clinical Competence, *David Newble & Dame Lesley Southgate*	30
■	Objectifying Skills Assessment: Bench Model Solutions, *Deepak Dath & Richard Reznick*	52
■	Communications Skills for Surgeons: the Need for Assessment, *Patricia Wilkie*	67
■	Proficiency Training for Space Flight, *Frank Hughes*	73
■	Challenges in Developing and Maintaining Skills and Proficiency, *Carolyn Huntoon & Arnauld Nicogossian*	81
■	The Clinical Link, *AW Goode*	91
■	The Opportunities for Virtual Reality and Simulation in the Training and Assessment of Technical Surgical Skills, *RJ Stone*	109
■	Assessment of Professional, Clinical and Surgical Skills in the Workplace, *Charles Galasko*	126

Surgical Competence

Challenges of assessment in training and practice

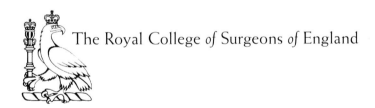

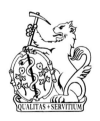

The Royal College *of* Surgeons *of* England

The
Smith & Nephew
Foundation

Published by the Royal College of Surgeons of England
Registered Charity No. 212808

35-43 Lincoln's Inn Fields
London WC2A 3PN
Tel: (0171) 405 3474
Fax: (0171) 831-9438
Internet: http://www.rcseng.ac.uk

First published 1999.
ISBN 0 902166 30 1

Typset by Chamberlain Dunn Associates, Richmond, England.
Printed by Holbrooks Printers Ltd, Portsmouth, England.

Foreword

For many years surgical competence has been assessed by the trainee needing to satisfactorily complete a specified number of years of training together with the passing of an examination in their surgical specialty. The examination varies among different specialties and countries but usually includes an MCQ component or some other form of written paper, a clinical examination and a viva voce. The examination tests knowledge of basic science and clinical skills but operative skills are rarely assessed. The content of the years of training is usually assessed by trainers and is subjective.

The question is now being asked as to whether subjective assessment of clinical training is adequate. If not, what objective methods of assessment could be employed on a regular basis to assess competence and eventually determine if the trainee has satisfactorily completed training? Is it correct to specify a fixed number of years of training? In many surgical specialties in the United Kingdom, six years are required as a specialist registrar; is it possible that some trainees may need only five years to reach the required competencies whereas others may take seven or eight years? If this is the case, what competencies are required by a surgeon and how should they be tested? Are examinations of the traditional kind really necessary at all?

This conference, generously sponsored by the Smith and Nephew Foundation and held in collaboration with The Royal College of Surgeons of England, examines the challenges posed by objective assessment of competence. The chapters that follow contain the substance of the presentations.

The College is delighted to be a partner with the Smith and Nephew Foundation in this important discussion and hopes that readers of this book will find much of interest and food for continued thought as the debate evolves. A robust method of competence assessment would revolutionise surgical training not only in the United Kingdom but in many other countries as well. I believe this conference will be a great stimulus to finding an eventual satisfactory outcome.

Barry Jackson
President, The Royal College of Surgeons of England

Why Do We Need to Assess Competence?

Sir Rex Richards FBA, FRS

Abstract

In the report of a task force on clinical academic careers, published by the CVCP in July 1997, one of many recommendations was '...the Royal Colleges should give serious consideration to establishing innovative procedures, other than written exit examinations, to assess clinical competence of candidates for the CCST, rather than just time spent.' The reasoning behind this recommendation to minimise disincentives to young doctors to follow an academic career involving research is explained. The advantages of reliable methods of assessing competence in both decision-making and in surgical skill are discussed. If appropriate simulators could be developed, it is suggested that they would be of very great help in selection and training.

I am a scientist by profession and am not medically qualified. Professor Galasko asked me to give this short introduction because I chaired an independent task force convened by the Committee of Vice Chancellors and Principals in the spring of 1996 to report on 'Clinical Academic Careers'. The task force consisted of seven eminent clinicians and five others who, though not medically qualified, had some serious interest in medical affairs.[1]

CLINICAL ACADEMIC CAREERS: THE NEED TO ASSESS COMPETENCE

A comprehensive questionnaire was completed by every medical and dental school in the United Kingdom, and a day visit was made by some members of the task force to every medical and dental school in England, Northern Ireland and Wales; the Scottish medical schools very generously agreed to meet us in Edinburgh. We reported in July 1997.[2]

One of many recommendations made in our report was:

> The Royal Colleges should give serious consideration to establishing innovative procedures, other than written exit examinations, to assess clinical competence of candidates for the CCST, rather than just time spent.

To describe the reasoning behind this recommendation I need to explain one of the major concerns of our report. 'Clinical academics' are members of a university, with a medical or dental degree and some specialist training, working in its medical or dental school; their activities are divided between patient care, teaching undergraduates, training young doctors and dentists for clinical accreditation, research, supervision of research, and, of course, the not inconsiderable administration and committee work which is nowadays required by the NHS and in higher education. Academics also play an important part in national (eg Royal Colleges, research councils, GMC, GDC, medical charities, BMA or BDA) and international (eg WHO and World Federations) medical and dental affairs.

Among all these activities, academics are expected to be particularly concerned with research into all aspects of medicine or dentistry, ranging from the basic science of discovery to the applied science of implementation, and encompassing work from the level of the molecule and the cell to the individual and the population. Such work ensures the continued development of new knowledge leading to improvements in healthcare. Of course, the NHS itself has had a long involvement in research, not only by supporting the work of academic staff in the medical and dental schools and in hospitals, but also by encouraging its own staff to engage in research projects if they are so minded. However, there is now a widespread perception that tighter management of the NHS has impaired the ability of consultants to continue research on the same scale as in the past. Resources are inevitably constrained, and they are now more precisely managed whichever NHS unit and purchaser or provider happens to be responsible for them. While this may in itself be laudable, a consequence is the apparent erosion of the scope for research driven by consultant initiative. This effect is reinforced by the increasingly technical nature of much current clinical research, which often requires access to high-cost equipment or specialist scientific support. One result of these changes is that clinical academics are becoming even more important as the 'research engine' of British medicine and dentistry.

Academic medicine and dentistry are serving two masters: in this case, the NHS and the universities. Both of these have been undergoing major, and ongoing, changes. Both are demanding greater efficiency, cost-effectiveness and more accountability. And both have introduced new education and training programs. The result is that staff in these areas work at a higher intensity with increased demands and expectations on them, and often with an increased administrative load. Clinical academics, working for both the NHS and the universities experience a double pressure and feel squeezed from both sides.

A major concern for clinical academics is therefore to establish the proper balance between their three main activities of service, research and education and training, and how this balance can be maintained. The division of effort between research, scholarship and teaching is, of course, faced by all academics, whatever the subject; but the addition of direct patient care, to which most clinical academics attach great importance, presents this issue in a particularly acute form.

Clinical academics are normally allocated sessions for each of these three main activities, but all of these are commonly exceeded; furthermore, we found overwhelming evidence that the service sessions were more often exceeded than the other allocations and that when under pressure, the research time was always the first to suffer.[3] This result is not at all surprising, for reasons set out in detail in our report, but pressure of such demanding work must make it difficult to maintain the momentum of research and to generate original and innovative ideas.

We were also concerned with medical training and the factors which acted as incentives or disincentives for clinicians to enter academic medicine.

We started work very soon after the Calman reforms of medical training were being brought into effect. Many specialist registrars welcomed the shorter and more structured training resulting from the reforms, but we noticed that some of the Specialist Advisory Committees of the Royal Colleges were very concerned that the shorter period of training might be insufficient to ensure that candidates for the CCST were fully competent to become consultants; this was particularly important for the procedural specialties which involve high skills and long practise. Indeed we met some young surgeons, in their last year before CCST, who were themselves far from happy that they had had sufficient opportunity to hone their operating skills. Some Specialist Advisory Committees therefore felt it necessary to prescribe more rigid curricula than in the past, with strict requirements for each procedure, feeling that the training in their speciality had now been reduced to an irreducible minimum.

While understanding the desire of the committees of the Royal Colleges to ensure that standards are maintained in the award of the CCST, many heads of departments were very concerned that new and rigid curricula discourage young clinicians from embarking on major research projects. Cases were cited to us where a specialist registrar taking time off for research found that his or her return to training did not always coincide with training timetables and he/she had to repeat some training, thus losing time and postponing still further the day when they might qualify for the CCST. Furthermore, our report goes on to say:

> It is argued that, as in all walks of life, even among the highly selected group of specialist registrars, there are significant variations in aptitude; some acquire skills more quickly than others. If the requirements for the CCST are now set at an irreducible minimum for the most skilled, how can we be sure that others, who may in the end be equally good, but learning more slowly, are ready to take responsibility? Alternatively, if the requirements are set for the slower learners, which we assume the current regulations are, is there not some way in which those moving more quickly could be allowed a shorter training period? It seems to us that certification based on competence, as well as or instead of just time and numbers of procedures completed, might be an alternative to be considered. We recognise the difficulty of devising a secure system of assessing competence, but feel that it is a goal worth pursuing; we also note that the GMC is now working on methods of assessment of performance. However, we are conscious that there are dangers of introducing written 'exit' examinations.

Doctors who are involved in research almost always do a certain amount of clinical service at the same time; they usually like doing it and value the experience they gain. Although it is envisaged that normally only one year of a period of research will be allowed to count towards the period of the SpR training, the additional clinical experience gained during two or three further years of research, with some clinical activity, would be valuable if a measure of competence as well as time was included in the requirements for the CCST.

It was these arguments which led the Task Force to make the above recommendation. What follows now are my own views, which I hope will be seen as those of a sympathetic outsider. I am sure that all these issues have been considered thoroughly by The Royal College of Surgeons, so hope that my comments do not seem naive.

SURGICAL COMPETENCE: THE NEED FOR MORE FORMAL ASSESSMENT

The medical Royal Colleges are justifiably proud of the long tradition of very high standards which they have maintained in the professions; their members and fellows are highly respected both at home and abroad. These standards have been upheld by close personal supervision of pupil by master and by traditional methods of examination, including written papers, observation on ward rounds, detailed study of clinical cases, and *viva voce* examinations. But the increasing demands of medical care in the NHS using procedures of ever increasing complexity, in hospitals where most patients are critically ill, place great physical, intellectual and emotional burdens on those responsible for patient care. These pressures must place strains on the process of medical education, and make us ask whether the rather informal methods which have worked so well in the past are appropriate for the future. Furthermore, there is an impression that some members of the public do not have the confidence and trust in the medical profession they used to have, and this has not been helped by some recent high profile cases. The question, therefore, is whether more formal methods of assessment are needed, particularly for operative skills which have not hitherto been tested objectively.

It is widely believed that about three-quarters of the skills required by a surgeon are intellectual and personal, and approximately one-quarter is based on technical competence, including manual dexterity and capacity for focused and sustained attention. Both of these are critically important. It is no good being able to handle tissue with great delicacy or to make beautiful sutures if you are not sure when and where to do it; equally, it is not much use knowing what needs to be done if it cannot be done skilfully.

Diagnostic and related skills

The intellectual and personal skills can be measured by well-established examination methods, provided that they are sufficiently structured to ensure consistency, relevance, and fairness; the traditional subjective methods which have long been used in universities have been much refined in many faculties over recent years to improve the objectivity and transparency of the judgements. Selection of staff for key positions in many other professions now often involves the use of techniques for formal assessment of various qualities and skills, which can be used and adapted with advantage in academic examining.[4][5] To ensure reliability and fairness, the various methods of testing require very careful preparation and co-ordination among different examiners. The Royal College of Surgeons initiated a very thorough study of objective methods for the selection of surgical trainees in 1987, based on the experience of the Royal Air Force in selection of aircrew over the past 50 years. As far as I am aware, however, these methods have not yet been adopted by the profession, so presumably there has been no attempt to validate them for surgical trainees. If such methods proved to be as valuable for aspiring surgeons as they are for aircrew selection, the additional cost would be rewarded amply by savings made on expensive training of ultimately unsuitable candidates.

Technical skills

The dexterity, eye-hand co-ordination and spatial skills of a surgeon seem to be much more difficult to assess.

Many surgeons believe it cannot be measured, that simulators measure skill at operating the simulator, and that this does not correlate well with high surgical skill in the handling of biological tissue. They believe that surgical dexterity can be assessed only by a skilled and experienced observer, and most say that they can tell a 'safe pair of hands' by watching a surgeon operating.

In the days when a young surgeon worked closely as an 'apprentice' through most of his or her training with a senior and experienced consultant surgeon, the judgement of the 'master' was no doubt pretty reliable. But this is surely not very satisfactory today when, in many hospitals, with the more structured training which has come with the Calman reforms, and with the period of training significantly reduced, a young surgeon is less likely to have senior colleagues who have watched him or her closely throughout their training.

On the other hand there are surgeons who believe that the need to find reliable methods of measuring surgical competence is an urgent matter.[6] It is argued that the results of surgical procedures are bound to vary with different hospitals and different surgeons, and that objective methods are needed to bring all up to the best.

Careful audit of results of procedures can be used to compare different centres, but the outcome must depend on case-mix, which is not the same in every centre. Some ways of allowing for this might be found. For example, it might be possible, though probably not popular, for one or two senior surgeons from one centre to exchange places for a limited period with surgeons from a centre which has been getting very different results.

Experienced surgeons could probably learn very quickly whether their techniques need updating or whether the differences in the results of the two centres are due mainly to a different case-mix or to other factors. ·

The audit method of comparing performance must, however, be imperfect, if only because it requires a prolonged period of study to produce statistical reliability, during which patients may be receiving less than the best treatment.

What other possibilities are there? Observation of procedural skill by more than one assessor using a structured scoring system has been shown to be more reliable than the subjective impressions now used,[7][8] but this is likely to be a cumbersome and expensive method unless the scoring system could be automated in some way.

One cannot help but be struck by the comparison of surgical competence and the qualities required of flying crew in the aviation industry. Both professions require high intellectual and personal skills, both require dexterity and good hand-eye co-ordination and both are responsible for the safety and indeed lives of their patients or passengers; the skills required are quite different, of course, but it cannot be denied that there are interesting parallels between them. Pilot error leading to the loss of an aircraft is a dramatic event involving enormous cost and, in some cases, dreadful loss of life, so the Air Force and the airline industry must select personnel for training very carefully, and carry out regular crew updates and assessments. They have been outstandingly successful in this respect, and perhaps there are important lessons which the medical profession could learn from them. Aircraft simulators have been brought to a remarkable degree of realism, and although the problems are very different, it is hard to believe that similarly realistic trainers could not be designed which would simulate many surgical procedures.

The possibility of measuring surgical skill by the use of simulators is now under study by Professor Darzi and his colleagues.[6] I am grateful to Professor Darzi for showing me some of his recent results, and it appears that even very simple simulators can provide data which correlate well with real surgical skill. It would surely be a good idea to stimulate the development of more complex and realistic simulators. Although this would require a very considerable investment of skill, knowledge and financial resources, which would have to be weighed up in a careful cost benefit analysis, the product could be of great assistance in selection, training and continuing education of surgeons. There could be considerable savings in training, and improved performance, and it is likely that there would be a very large market world-wide for such a simulator. So at what stage(s) would simulators be valuable?

Stages of assessment

There appear to me to be three main stages where assessment would be of advantage. The first is at the selection of surgical trainees. Dexterity and hand-eye co-ordination do not always go with intellectual ability, and I know from my own experience that even among the most intellectually able young research collaborators, there can be a wide range of manual dexterity, varying from people who have natural skills and can perform difficult laboratory tasks with ease, to those who seem to get into difficulties with the most simple operations. Similar variations must also occur among doctors; no doubt those who have really poor manual dexterity are self deselected or come to notice at a very early stage and are discouraged from embarking on surgical training. But is there a possibility that some young surgical trainees are allowed to go forward until their limitations become obvious? If so, his or her mentors must then be faced with the unenviable task of explaining the situation to them and helping them to cope with the personal trauma involved by steering them into some other branch of medicine; and there must be marginal cases where the trainee would be given the benefit of the doubt and perhaps proceed into a profession in which he or she will never excel.

Perhaps this is a situation where a simulator could be designed which would be reliable enough to filter out really unsuitable candidates at an early stage; its cost could be set against the considerable cost of surgical training and the personal cost to an able doctor who proves not to have the particular qualities required of a surgeon. Simple mechanical simulators of some basic surgical procedures are already widely used and have proved very helpful to aspiring surgeons, though they are mainly very limited in scope.

The next stage of assessment might be at the point of certification; it would be just one factor to be taken into account in the process of measurement of competence to decide whether the candidate is ready to be considered for a consultancy. This would require simulators of much greater sophistication. The cost would have to be balanced against the value of the simulators during training, which might be very considerable if they were truly realistic, and the confidence it would give in the final assessment, which would include the very wide range of measures of attributes which surgeons require. It may well be that a simulator would never be able to mimic the many and varied technical problems faced by a surgeon during an operation, but even if it provided practice in some important skills, and could be placed in an environment where the various stressful and distracting incidents which occur in real operating theatres from time to time could be reproduced, it could be of enormous benefit to surgeons, whether they are trainees or experienced practitioners.

If appropriately sophisticated simulators could be developed, they might prove to be very valuable for in-service training (CME) and to assist surgeons to maintain their skills in procedures which, by virtue of their position, they have to face only occasionally in the operating theatre.

Finally, I am informed that airline aircrew are required to pass a medical examination at regular intervals; so far as I am aware, this is not customary for surgeons except on appointment.

CONCLUSIONS

So why should we seek reliable means to assess surgical competence?

■ Examination methods which are sufficiently structured to ensure consistency, relevance and fairness, together with tests of dexterity, would ensure that candidates for surgical training have sufficient promise to justify the very considerable cost of training.

■ Appropriate simulators would provide opportunities for trainee surgeons to learn basic skills by repeating procedures as frequently as they think necessary without having to wait for appropriate patients.

■ Simulators as well as other assessment methods could be used to check that a surgeon's competence is improving during training.

■ Simulators could be used to provide part of the information required to assess competence for the CCST, and regularly thereafter to maintain and revise skills. They could be placed in an environment to reproduce the stressful and distracting events which often occur in a real operating theatre.

■ Assessment of competence would help clinical academics to fit in their research and service work in the most effective way for every individual.

■ Better outcomes for patients could be expected.

■ The profession and the public would have greater confidence in the ability of surgical teams.

■ If suitable simulators are to be developed, the initial cost would be very considerable, and would have to be balanced against factors mentioned above.

ACKNOWLEDGEMENTS

I am very grateful to a number of surgeons who very generously made time to talk to me about surgical practice and training. Professor Darzi and his colleagues at St Mary's Hospital were also kind enough to show me some demonstrations of their studies using laparoscopic simulators. The views I have expressed here are those I have formed after these discussions.

References

1.   The members of the Task Force were: Sir Rex Richards FBA, FRS (Chairman); Professor Sir Michael Bond FRCPsych, FRCP Glas, FRCSE; Professor Robert Burgess BA, PhD; Dame Fiona Caldicott FRCPsych, FRCP FRCPI, FRCGP; Professor Sir David Carter FRCSE, FRCSGlas; Mr John Cooper BA, MBA, AHA; Sir Christopher France GCB; Dr David Gordon MB, FRCP; Professor Ann-Louise Kinmonth MD, MSc, FRCPG, FRCP, FRCCH; Professor Sir Keith Peter FRCP, FRS; Sir Derek Roberts Feng, FinstP, FRS; Professor Colin Smith BDS, PhD, LDS, FRCPath.

2.   Clinical Academic Careers. *CVCP*; 1997. p 104.

3.   Goldacre M, Stear S, Richards R, Sidebottom E. Junior doctors' views about careers in academic medicine. *Medical Education* 1999; 33:318-326.

4.   See for example: Gough MH. In: Morris PJ, Malt RJ, eds. *Oxford Textbook of Surgery*. 2nd ed. Oxford: Oxford University Press. p 2751.

5.   Bulstrode C, Hunt V. *Examining Consultants*. Oxford: The SUMIT Project; 1997.

6.   Darzi A, Smith S, Taffinder N. Assessing operative skill. *BMJ* 1999; 318:887.

7.   Martin JA, Regehr G, Reznick R, MacRae H, Murnaghan J, Hutchison C, et al. Objective structured assessment of technical skill (OSATS) for surgical residents. *Br J Surg* 1997; 84:273.

8.   Faulkner H, Regehr G, Martin J, Reznick R. Validation of an objective structured assessment of technical skill for surgical residents. *Acad Med* 1996; 71: 1363.

Clinical Performance in the National Health Service

Professor Liam J Donaldson MSc MD FRCS(Ed) FRCP FFPHM

Chief Medical Officer, Department of Health

Abstract

The exercise of professional judgement and the development of clinical skills are important determinants of the quality of surgical care provided to patients. In turn, the way in which high standards in these areas are assured and developed within an organisational setting is a key function of a modern health service.

The National Health Service (NHS) in Britain is in its fifty-second year of existence. Over this time, the approach taken to ensuring good performance of services has gradually evolved from one which was largely based on implicit assumptions about maintaining standards to a managed system in which there is much greater clarity about what is expected and a more explicit accountability for achieving results.

This chapter sets out an overview of clinical performance in the NHS – how it has developed, what some of the problems have been and how they are currently being addressed. Although the account is set primarily in a United Kingdom context, many of the issues will be common to other healthcare systems.

PRIORITY-SETTING AND PERFORMANCE MANAGEMENT

The process of delivery of care through the NHS begins with the creation of policies, strategies and targets at national and local level which are operationalised in area-wide plans (called health improvement programs) and delivered by a range of providers of services in primary care, in hospitals and in the community.

The range of inputs to this planning process is very diverse and includes national and local assessments of need, the views of expert bodies, the review of health information, awareness of new opportunities arising from developments in medical technology, and evidence of clinical effectiveness arising from research. Each year, a statement of priorities is issued by the NHS Executive[1] (the national strategic level of NHS management) to all health authorities, primary care groups and Trusts and NHS Trusts (the main bodies responsible for planning and delivering healthcare at local level). In the last few years this statement of priorities has been addressed jointly to the health service and local authorities, in recognition of the importance of the latter in promoting the health of local communities and caring for people with long-term and chronic diseases.

This broad statement of priorities at national level is then worked up by all relevant agencies (health and non-health) into a health improvement program which formulates more detailed priorities, targets and plans to maintain and improve healthcare for local communities. The health improvement program is the main determinant of how the health service is resourced around the country.

The assessment of the performance of the NHS against its objectives set out in the various priority statements and plans take place at all levels of the service. A nationally set framework lays out a basis against which the success of the NHS can be judged broadly (Table 1).

Table 1.   **National performance measures**

- health improvement
- fair access
- effective delivery of healthcare
- efficiency
- patient and carer experience
- health outcomes

Source: *The New NHS: Modern and Dependable* [2]

At local level, health authorities monitor the health improvement programs which have been agreed. Within health organisations providing care – for example NHS Trusts, hospitals or primary care groups – managers, including clinician managers, ensure that the agreed levels of services and performance targets are delivered. The eight regional offices of the NHS Executive which cover England also ensure that the strategies of the NHS are delivered to plan.

In practice, the management of the performance of surgical and other services is much more complex than this basic description of the process suggests. This is because in a highly devolved service (over 1,000 individual NHS organisations in England) with considerable local autonomy, achieving a consistent standard is difficult. Moreover, priorities once set are subject to change as funding and workload pressures develop in a particular year. Thus, pre-agreed waiting time targets for planned surgical operations might be threatened by a surge of emergency admissions due (say) to a winter influenza epidemic.

With this general context, and the way in which the performance of NHS services is managed, the remainder of the chapter concentrates on service performance in relation to the delivery of healthcare quality.

CLINICAL QUALITY: AN EVOLVING CONCEPT

At the heart of any consideration of clinical quality lie three elements: the philosophy or concept of quality which is being pursued; the methodologies which are being used to assure or improve quality; and the measures which are used to assess it.

Over time, there has been a huge diversity in all three of these elements within the different approaches that have been taken. Whilst attempts to address quality in the provision of clinical services, including surgical practice, has a long history, viewed internationally the impetus to address healthcare quality within organised health services dates mainly from the 1960s.

The concept of quality set out by the North American health services researcher Donabedian[3] is one which has been influential for over 30 years. In this, quality is seen as comprising three strands – structures, processes and outcomes. Donabedian used the term 'structure' to include the amount and nature of staff and facilities available to a health service. Process on the other hand was described as that aspect of quality assessed by what is done for and to the patient. Good quality in process terms can be judged against best practice guidelines. The third component of the triad is the outcome of the healthcare episode for the patient. Does he or she get better? Were there surgical complications? Is the patient satisfied with their surgical care? Do they survive?

Whilst the outcome of care is the final arbiter of quality, it is the interrelationship between the structure, process and outcome which is important and which is not always fully understood. Thus, good outcomes of vascular surgery will depend on the numbers and skill of the surgeons in a team, and the specialised facilities available to them as well as how the team organises its work and applies best practice techniques. Poor outcomes might result from inadequate staffing levels and infrastructure (ie structural deficit) or they might arise from poorly organised services and inappropriate clinical policies, even in a well-staffed, well-equipped service (ie weak process).

During the first two decades of the NHS, the main focus of systematic quality improvement was on structural aspects. Much of the planning to improve services was based on ideas of 'norms' (eg desired numbers of surgeons or hospital beds per head of population). At this time, the concept of quality was largely implicit. It was believed that if healthcare facilities were adequately staffed by highly skilled, well-trained staff, sufficiently supported by the right technology, then high-quality care would be assured.

Over time this position changed gradually within the NHS. By the 1980s, management was becoming established with a move away from the diffuse notion of administration of health services towards clear accountability for the performance of every health organisation within the system. The appointment of general managers[4] or chief executives was gradually followed by the establishment of clinical directorates through which surgeons and other clinicians held budgets for their own services and participated in the corporate management of the hospital. This shift towards managed health organisations was initially viewed with suspicion by clinicians but gradually embraced so that by the mid-1990s there were few hospitals in which explicit clinical management structures were not in place. Indeed, in some of the 'big city' teaching hospitals, the budget of a single clinical directorate, say surgical services, was bigger than that of a whole general hospital in one of the surrounding smaller towns.

These developments led to the idea that the structure of the NHS could be re-designed to create incentives for greater efficiency and improved quality. Therefore, in the early 1990s, an internal market was established[5] in which the roles of different bodies within the NHS were redefined as either 'purchasers' of services (health authorities and general practice fundholders) or 'providers' of services (hospitals, community health services, ambulance services) which eventually became NHS Trusts. In theory, it was held that the internal market would simulate the behaviours of a real market and raise quality whilst driving out inefficiencies. Purchasers would use their budgets to ensure that contracts were placed where higher quality and best value could be achieved whilst providers of service would compete to do better than their peers in order to secure a share of these budgets.

This concept of quality improvement remained controversial and many professional staff working in the NHS and apparently the general public did not see its claimed benefits being realised in day-to-day services.

The new Labour government which came to power in Britain in the spring of 1997 dismantled the internal market and replaced it with a system based on partnership and collaboration, not competition.[2]

Relatively, little progress has been made in developing routinely available measures of healthcare quality. Waiting times for surgical operations and out-patient consultation is an important measure of a health service's performance but it gives no insight into more fundamental aspects of quality. Aside from research studies and projects run in individual services, hardly any data on clinical outcome are available for day-to-day assessment of service performance. The development of outcome indicators has been largely a research and professional activity. Indeed, throughout the whole of this period of evolving health policy in relation to performance and quality of health services, initiatives by professional bodies to improve standards of practice have continued. These have taken a variety of forms. Participation in clinical audit has been a contractual responsibility since the early 1990s[6] for consultants working in the NHS although it was commonly practised before that time. Major national audits have been helpful in highlighting weaknesses in the performance or organisation of services and the Confidential Enquiry into Perioperative Deaths (CEPOD)[7] is a good example. Professional bodies continue to produce expert reports which draw attention to problems with the performance of services or of the need for change in the care of patients with specific diseases or in particular areas of specialist practice.[8]

A major focus of professionally led quality improvement activity in the 1990s has been the production of guidelines to encourage the adoption of best practice. This flowed from the recognition that the transfer of knowledge gained from research about therapeutic effectiveness into routine clinical practice was a slow process.[9] It also became clear that variation in medical practice far in excess of what would be expected by differences in morbidity was a feature of many healthcare systems. Guidelines do improve clinical performance but the size of the improvement varies considerably.[10] A balance has to be struck between the authority of guidelines produced by national or international experts and the greater likelihood of ownership if guidelines are derived locally. However, the two essential criteria for practice guidelines to improve clinical performance is that they accord with research evidence and that they are complied with by clinicians.[11]

Another approach is to set explicit standards for practice in an area of care against which the performance of the service and individuals within it can be assessed.[12]

A new paradigm of clinical practice emerged from this awareness of the importance of shifting from research into practice. This philosophy of evidence-based medicine rapidly became international in its scope[13] and now underpins much of the modern approach to practice (Figure 1).

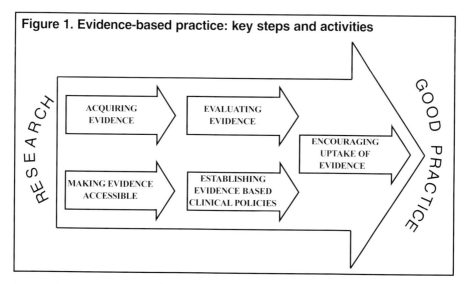

Figure 1. Evidence-based practice: key steps and activities

RESEARCH

ACQUIRING EVIDENCE

EVALUATING EVIDENCE

ENCOURAGING UPTAKE OF EVIDENCE

MAKING EVIDENCE ACCESSIBLE

ESTABLISHING EVIDENCE BASED CLINICAL POLICIES

GOOD PRACTICE

Source: Donaldson LJ, Donaldson RJ. *Essential Public Health*. London: Petroc Press, 1999 (in press).

A NEW INTEGRATED APPROACH TO QUALITY

As part of its new policies for the NHS in the late 1990s, the Labour government placed a duty of quality on every health organisation within the NHS. At a local level this is translated into clinical governance defined as:[14]

> Clinical governance is a framework through which NHS organisations are accountable for continuously improving the quality of their services and safeguarding high standards of care by creating an environment in which excellence in clinical care will flourish.

Clinical governance is essentially an organisational concept aimed at ensuring that every health organisation creates the culture, the systems and the support mechanisms so that good clinical performance will be the norm and so that quality improvement will be a key part of routine clinical practice.[15, 16, 17]

Placing a duty of quality on the NHS – a duty not just to assure high standards but to improve year on year – is a bold and imaginative challenge and an approach which attempts to reset the balance in which financial and workload targets have dominated management thinking in the NHS.[18]

The local duty of quality is reinforced by the creation of two new national bodies – the National Institute for Clinical Excellence (NICE) which will set standards, and the Commission for Health Improvement which will inspect local clinical governance arrangements and investigate where services appear to be failing (Figure 2).

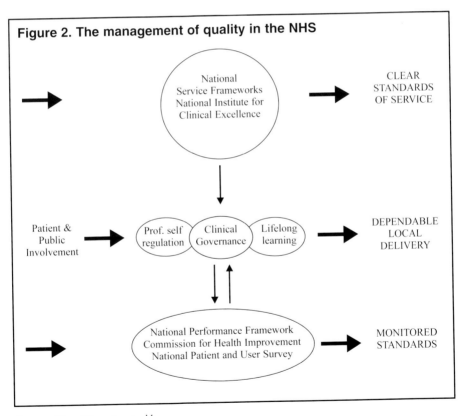

Figure 2. The management of quality in the NHS

National Service Frameworks National Institute for Clinical Excellence

CLEAR STANDARDS OF SERVICE

Patient & Public Involvement

Prof. self regulation / Clinical Governance / Lifelong learning

DEPENDABLE LOCAL DELIVERY

National Performance Framework Commission for Health Improvement National Patient and User Survey

MONITORED STANDARDS

Source: *First Class Service*[14]

Clinical governance seeks to create a focus on quality improvement in every health organisation, every service and every clinical team which will eventually lead to a step up in the quality of care closer to that provided in the best performing services and a shift in the quality curve to the right (Figure 3).[15]

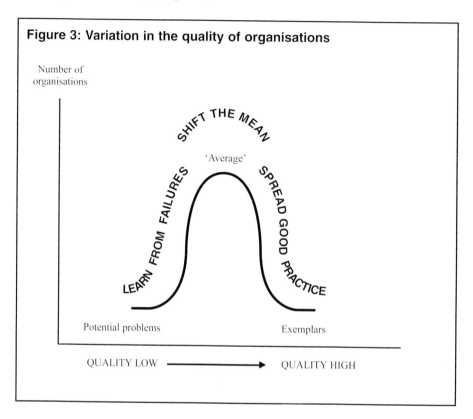

Figure 3: Variation in the quality of organisations

A NEW CONCEPT OF CLINICAL ACCOUNTABILITY

The shift towards a more managed system of care in the NHS of the 1980s and 1990s and the new statutory duty of quality introduced in the late 1990s, have implications for the traditional concept of clinical accountability. For most of the lifetime of the NHS, the accountability of a surgeon or other clinician was to his or her individual patients and to a broad professional code. Practice was largely self-determined. Today, a doctor has a range of new accountabilities arising, for example, from tighter more explicit professional standards, a duty to participate in continuing professional development and to the corporate goals of the service in which they work (Figure 4).

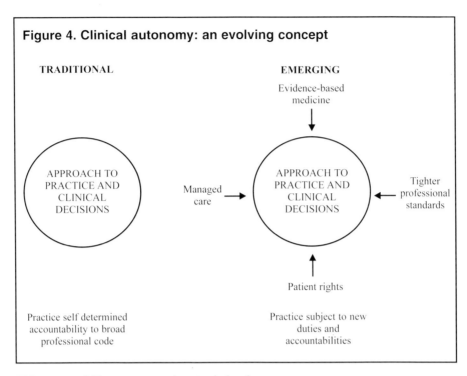

Figure 4. Clinical autonomy: an evolving concept

TRADITIONAL

EMERGING

Evidence-based
medicine

APPROACH TO
PRACTICE AND
CLINICAL
DECISIONS

Managed
care

APPROACH TO
PRACTICE AND
CLINICAL
DECISIONS

Tighter
professional
standards

Patient rights

Practice self determined
accountability to broad
professional code

Practice subject to new
duties and
accountabilities

This accountability operates at three main levels:

■ first, the accountability of the individual professional for the quality of his or her own work;

■ secondly, the accountability of the professional within an organisation in which he or she works. An accountability, for example to participate in the clinical governance program as it develops; and

■ thirdly, their accountability as a member of the senior staff of the organisation, shared with others for that organisation's performance or more widely for local services.

Ultimately, it is likely that there will be a formal realignment and reshaping of traditional professional autonomy in the light of these developments and changes.

POOR PRACTITIONER PERFORMANCE

The question of poor performance on the part of individual clinical practitioners has become the subject of public and professional concern during the late 1990s. On the surface, the NHS has had long-standing disciplinary procedures for dealing with incompetence or professional misconduct whilst the main body regulating medical practice in the United Kingdom – the General Medical Council – has powers to deal with problems of ill health, serious professional misconduct and (more recently) poor performance which arise amongst registered medical practitioners.[19]

Below the surface, over most of the lifetime of the NHS, this has remained a taboo subject for a whole variety of reasons, just some of which are: a tendency within the medical profession in the past to tolerate deviant behaviour; a reluctance of doctors to criticise their colleagues or give evidence against them in a formal setting because of feelings of disloyalty or a fear of being sued; ambiguity about where to draw the line between acceptable and unacceptable practice.[20] [21] There are other institutional reasons why the problem has not been well-addressed in the past. Procedures within the NHS have been heavily weighted towards disciplinary approaches with a strong legalistic basis. As a result, employers seem to have found such procedures daunting and hence were reluctant to use them except as a last resort. Doctors with problems have undoubtedly continued in practice when they should not have done so.

During the 1990s, an increasing number of cases wherein a doctor's practice had given rise to concern came to public attention. Typically, there was extensive media coverage, the doctor was suspended for a long period of time (with no clear end-point in sight), the issues were too complex for local managers to unravel, and there were legal challenges by lawyers representing patients or doctors. All too often, the consequences were serious loss of public confidence in a local service, low morale in the clinical department concerned, great expense and a disproportionate amount of time spent by the management of the hospital, leading to further press stories and legal representations. For the surgeon, the opportunity for re-education or re-skilling is often lost permanently.

Failure to meet acceptable standards of performance can be manifest in many ways.[19] Poor clinical performance can be associated, for example, with errors or delays in making diagnoses, with inappropriate use of tests or treatments, and with technical errors in the performance of a procedure. Other problems may have to do with behaviour: poor communication with patients, the inability to work as a member of a team, rude and disruptive conduct. In other cases, there may be underlying ill-health problems which contribute to a failure to perform to a good standard.

In the late 1990s one case in particular can be regarded as a watershed in the history of poor clinical performance in the NHS.[22] The Bristol children's heart surgery service from which two doctors were struck off the medical register and one blamed for operating on children following consideration of the accusations by the General Medical Council.

Ultimately, the focus of attention when dealing with poor clinical performance must be on prevention and early detection as much as on establishing mechanisms to deal with the consequences. To this end, the General Medical Council has put forward proposals to 'revalidate' doctors' licences to practise every five years. In the NHS, key elements of this will be strong programs of training, continuing professional development, appraisal and good systems of data to assess performance.

Consideration of the question of poor individual performance must not overlook the need to acknowledge the importance of a system's perspective to service failure. In other sectors (eg: manufacturing, airline industry, military) it has long been recognised that some environments are at risk of error which can lead to disaster. The healthcare sector has been slow to appreciate this but it is now being taken seriously.[23][24]

CONCLUSIONS

Ensuring good performance of the surgical and other services provided by the NHS in Britain has shifted from a long-standing emphasis on workload and efficiency targets to one in which there is now a statutory duty to assure and improve quality. The concept of clinical governance places a clear accountability on each health organisation in the country to deliver quality goals by creating a culture in which clinical excellence will flourish.

It brings with it a new more explicit form of clinical accountability and a responsibility for a more robust approach to poor individual practitioner performance than has existed in the past.

A strong and constructive partnership between the medical profession, the NHS and government will be essential if the full potential of this new quality agenda is to be realised into the next century.

References

1.   Department of Health. Modernising Health and Social Services National Priorities Guidance 1999/00 and 2001/02. *Health Service Circular.* London: 1998/159.

2.   Department of Health. *The New NHS: Modern, Dependable*. The Stationery Office. London: 1997, (Cm 3807).

3.   Donabedian A. Evaluating the quality of medical care. *Milbank Memorial Fund Quarterly* 1966; 4: 166-206.

4.   Department of Health and Social Security Griffiths R. *NHS Management Enquiry.*
        London: 1983.

5.   Department of Health. *Working for Patients.* The Stationery Office. London: (Cm 555).

6.   Department of Health. *Medical audit in the hospital and community services. Health
        Circular* 91(2). The Stationery Office. London: 1991.

7.   National Confidential Enquiry into Perioperative Deaths. Gray AJG, Hoile RW, Ingram
        GS, Sherry KM, compilers. *The Report of the National Confidential Enquiry into
        Perioperative Deaths 1996/1997* (1 April 1996 to 31 March 1997). London: 1998.

8.   The Royal College of Surgeons of England. *The Report of the Working Party on the
        Management of Patients with Head Injuries.* London: 1999.

9.   Eddy DM. Clinical policies and the quality of clinical practice. *N Engl J Med* 1982;
        307: 343-347.

10.   Grimshaw JM, Russell IT. Effect of clinical guidelines on medical practice: a systematic
        review of rigorous evaluations. *Lancet* 1993; 342:1317-1322.

11.   Donaldson LJ, Hayes JH, Barton AG, Howel D, Hawthorne M. Impact of clinical prac-
        tice guidelines on clinicians' behaviour: tonsillectomy in children. *The Journal of
        Otolaryngology* 1999; 28: 24-30.

12.   Irvine DH, Donaldson LJ. Quality and standards in healthcare. *Proceedings of the Royal
        Society of Edinburgh* 1993; 101B: 1-30.

13.   Evidence-based Medicine Working Group. Evidence-based medicine: a new approach
        to teaching the practice of medicine. *JAMA* 1992; 268: 2420-2425.

14.   Department of Health. A First Class Service: Quality in the New NHS. London: 1998
        (*Health Service Circular:* HSC(98)113).

15.   Scally G, Donaldson LJ. Clinical governance and the drive for quality improvement in
        the new NHS in England. *BMJ* 1998; 317: 61-65.

16.   Donaldson LJ, Gray JAM. Clinical governance: a quality duty for health organisations.
        Quality in Health Care 1988; 7(suppl 1): S37-S44.

17.   Ayres PJ, Wright J, Donaldson LJ. Achieving clinical effectiveness: the new world of
        Clinical Governance. *Clinician in Management* 1998; 7:106-111.

18.   Donaldson LJ. Clinical Governance: a new statutory duty for quality improvement.
        Journal of Epidemiology and Community Health 1998, 52:73-74.

19.   Donaldson LJ. Doctors with problems in an NHS workforce. *BMJ* 1994; 308:1277-1282.

20.   Donaldson LJ. (1997) Doctors with problems in a hospital workforce. In: Lens P, Wal G van der (eds) *Problem Doctors: A Conspiracy of silence*. Amsterdam: 10S Press, 1997.

21.   Donaldson LJ. Facing up to the problem of the poorly performing doctor. *Student BMJ* 1996; 4: 276-7.

22.   Smith R. Regulation of doctors and the Bristol inquiry. Both need to be credible to both the public and doctors. *BMJ* 1998; 317: 1539-40.

23.   Donaldson LJ. Medical mishaps: a managerial perspective. In: Rosenthal M M, Mulcahy L and Lloyd-Bostock S (eds). *Medical Mishaps: Pieces of the Puzzle*. Open University Press, February 1999.

24.   Leape L. A systems analysis approach to medical error. *Journal of Evaluation in Clinical Practice* 1997; 3: 213-222.

The Principles and Practice of Assessing Clinical Competence

David Newble BSc (Hons), MD, FRACP, DipEd

Professor and Head, Department of Medical Education, University of Sheffield.

Lesley Southgate DBE, M Clin Sci, FRCP, FRCGP, F Med Sci

Professor of Primary Care and Medical Education, Centre for Health Informatics and Multiprofessional Education, Royal Free and University College Medical School

Abstract

In the UK, medical schools, colleges and the GMC all have the responsibility to develop and run 'high stakes' assessments of clinical competence. These are expected to be of high quality and meet internationally credible standards of validity and reliability.

This chapter describes literature-based guidelines which can be used by designers of clinical assessments. It sets out steps on how to determine the purpose; define what is to be tested; select test methods; address issues of administration and scoring; and set standards. This section is followed by three case studies drawn from the experience of the authors, which illustrate how these guidelines have been applied in practice.

INTRODUCTION

Medical schools and colleges have traditionally been the main organisations in the UK responsible for assessing competence during and at the conclusion of undergraduate and postgraduate education. More recently, the introduction of procedures to identify and assess potentially under-performing doctors, the assessment of the competence of doctors coming to the UK from other countries, and the move to re-certify or revalidate the competence of doctors over their practising lifetime has been accompanied by a change in the involvement of the General Medical Council (GMC) assessing the competence of doctors on the UK Register. In common with licensing bodies internationally, the GMC has moved from a reactive to a proactive stance.[1] Many of these procedures can be seen as 'high stakes' assessments from the perspective both of those being assessed and of the community. As such, there are expectations that they be of high quality, meeting internationally credible standards of validity and reliability. Most organisations responsible for such assessments have recognised that many of the procedures and decision-making processes used in the past have left much to be desired and are moving rapidly to meet acceptable evidence-based standards of testing.

This chapter will outline a set of literature-based guidelines which can be used by all designers of clinical assessments which, if followed, will do much to ensure their quality. Case studies will then be described which will demonstrate in a practical way how these guidelines have been used in practice. The main focus will be on formal summative assessment approaches which are used for certification purposes rather than formative approaches used during training or continuing professional development. Nevertheless, it is important to recognise the close inter-relationship of formative and summative approaches in any comprehensive set of assessment procedures. It is also important to remember that we are unlikely ever to be able to assess all the competencies and attributes essential to good practice in an examination. Some can only be assessed directly in the real practice setting. The growing recognition of the need for more valid and reliable procedures of this type is an area of debate and active research, and will be enhanced by the imperatives of revalidation and clinical governance.

GUIDELINES FOR ASSESSING CLINICAL COMPETENCE

This section is based on work arising from the Fifth Cambridge Conference on Medical Education held in Adelaide, Australia in 1991.[2] [3] The guidelines are a reflection of the literature and of the views and experiences of international experts on clinical assessment. They consist of a set of processes and sequential steps which should be followed if a rational approach to test development is to be achieved (see Figure 1). They also provide a comprehensive set of references relevant to this section of the chapter.

Determine the purpose

The purpose of the assessment must be quite clear. The procedures chosen could vary quite considerably depending on the purpose. Institutions often attempt to use one form of assessment for more than one purpose and this is usually a mistake. Examples include using the results of objective tests (MCQs) to make predictions about clinical competence; using tests developed for formative purposes to make summative decisions or vice-versa; and attempting to use the same procedures and results to make pass/fail or competency-based decisions and ranking or distinction decisions.

Define what is to be tested

Being clear on what is to be tested is fundamental to establishing the content validity of the procedure. It is the way of guiding the definition of the expected competence from which a representative sample has to be drawn during the assessment. Without this other important attributes, such as reliability, are of little consequence.

Three steps are involved:

Step 1: Identify the desired level of resolution

The task of identifying the content of a clinical competence assessment should be based on the clinical problems relevant to the area of interest (eg those to be faced by a PRHO for a final-year medical student examination). There should be a rational and systematic approach to identifying the problems which may include the collated opinions of experts and analysis of workplace situations. The problems may be stated as presenting complaints (eg abdominal pain; shortness of breath; difficulty with micturition) or may be framed as core conditions (eg periphero-vascular disease; bowel obstruction). It may also be desirable to include a range of expected practical skills common to managing many problems (eg suturing; IV insertion). In compiling the list of problems, considerations such as frequency, importance and severity must be taken into account.

Step 2: Define the clinical tasks within each problem that must be performed competently

In this context, the term 'clinical tasks' refers to actions that are specific to a particular clinical problem. They will comprise a range of knowledge and skills that are essential if the problem is to be satisfactorily managed. These must be defined in

Figure 1. Guidelines for assessing clinical competence

Determine The Purpose

Defining What Is To Be Tested
Step 1: Identify the clinical desired level of resolution
Step 2: For each problem, define the clinical tasks at which students are expected to be competent
Step 3: Prepare a blueprint to guide the selection of problems to be included in the assessment procedure

Selecting Test Methods
Step 1: Select test methods that are most appropriate to the clinical tasks being assessed
Step 2: Let the clinical task dictate the method by which it is tested
Step 3: Recognise the practical constraints on selecting optimal examination methods

Addressing Issues of Test Administration and Scoring
Step 1: Decide on the level of efficiency needed in the particular testing environment
Step 2: Decide how the student's performance is to be recorded or captured
Step 3: Determine a method to assign scores to the cases and/or elements within cases
Step 4: Take appropriate steps to ensure that the test provides an unbiased measure of performance
Step 5: Evaluate the need for equating scores across different examinations
Step 6: Review the procedure to ensure that trivialisation has not occurred

Setting Standards for Performance
Step 1: Determine the type of standard desired and an appropriate standard-setting method
Step 2: Develop procedure for effectively communicating the results of the test

specific terms and at a level of resolution appropriate to the expected performance of the student or doctor concerned. For example, for the problem of acute abdominal pain, a student or PRHO would be expected only to diagnose acute appendicitis while the surgical SpR would in addition be expected to perform the appendectomy.

Research on assessing clinical competence has established very clearly that valid and reliable results will only occur if a wide sampling of problems and tasks is undertaken. This has important consequences for the length of assessment procedures.

Step 3: Prepare a blueprint to guide problem/task selection

A comprehensive content and competencies blueprint should be developed for any assessment procedure. In some situations this can be quite simple and unidimensional, such as assigning weights to various disciplines in an examination. In other situations, particularly those representing high stakes assessments of competence such as final year student examinations and College examinations, a more complex, multidimension 'grid' will be required. One dimension will represent the problems, the other will reflect categories of competence such as data-gathering, diagnosis, investigation, management, communication, technical skills and so on. The blueprint will then indicate the specific and critical tasks embedded in the problems which should be tested.

Blueprints form the basis on which the sample for testing is selected. Ideally, this should be a random sample of enough problems/tasks and all competence categories to ensure the validity and reliability of the assessment. On the other hand, this procedure should not lead to the testing of a large number of isolated bits of information or skill. They should all be referenced to and embedded in important and relevant problems which the person being assessed should be competent to deal with.

These steps, though initially time-consuming, provide a practical approach to establishing the most important component of a good assessment procedure – a high-level of content validity. The subsequent use of elegant test methods, computerised scoring systems or sophisticated analytic procedures cannot compensate for a failure at this stage.

Selecting test methods

There is now a wide range of test methods available for use in assessing clinical competence.[4] These cannot be discussed in detail. This section discusses the importance of being aware of the toolkit of methods available and of selecting the methods which best match the content to be tested.

Three steps should be followed:

Step 1: Select methods most appropriate for the clinical tasks to be assessed

Over the last 20 years, strenuous efforts have been made to develop forms of assessment which are more valid, efficient and reliable than traditional forms. These have included written and computer-based patient management problems (PMPs); multi-station examinations like the objective structured clinical examination (OSCE) and standardised patient (SP)-based examinations; and new written tests such as extended matching and key feature approaches. Each has its limitations, particularly those involving performance-based components, the most frustrating being the prolonged testing time required to achieve acceptable levels of reliability for high stakes assessment. This phenomenon is variously called case specificity, content specificity or problem specificity. It represents the inherent nature of dealing with clinical problems in which performance on one problem is a very poor predictor of performance on another problem.

Selecting the method relates to the purpose of the overall test or a sub-component. For assessing some aspects of diagnostic skill or the ability to order investigations, a written or computer-based form may suffice and if so, assessment may be completed quite efficiently. Where clinical skills are to be assessed, such as history-taking, patient education, physical examination and technical procedures, this can only be achieved validly using multiple observation of performance on real or simulated patients, or sometimes on manikins or models.

Step 2: Let the clinical task dictate the method by which it is tested

Letting the purpose determine the method seems self-evident. However, in the real world, selection of methods is often arbitrary and based as much on convenience or tradition as on a rational match with purpose. For example, tests used for certifying competence to practice have sometimes relied exclusively on multiple-choice tests. Clearly, many important aspects of competence could not be assessed using this test format. There is a move to higher fidelity formats with greater scope for testing a wider range of competencies. However, no one method is capable of measuring all components and any comprehensive assessment procedure will consist of more than one test method.

Step 3: Recognise the practical constraints on selecting optimal test methods

Usually it is not possible to achieve an ideal match between the clinical tasks being posed and the method of assessments. Constraints include time available for testing, resources for development and conducting the assessment (eg. money, examiners, organisers, patients, facilities), the measurement characteristics of the available methods, and the acceptability of the ideal approach to the commissioning organisation, the examiners and the profession.

Addressing issues of test administration and scoring

Administrative problems, such as the need to test large numbers of candidates, have often led to the overuse of methods which are efficient but not necessarily appropriate (eg multiple-choice tests). This situation is changing as organisations are facing up to the challenge of broadening the base of testing. The introduction of computer-based testing and multi-site, multi-station examinations are examples of this.[5] [6] The additional practical problems relating to issues such as security, training and consistency across sites are considerable when there are large numbers of candidates to be assessed.

Six steps should be followed:
Step 1: Decide on the required level of efficiency

Previously, we indicated that a valid assessment of clinical competence will usually require the use of more than one test method – generally a written test and a clinical test. Efficiency is increased if these could be arranged so that the more efficient test is administered first and the less efficient test is undertaken only by those passing the first hurdle. There are potential dangers in this strategy if both components are not linked to the same blueprint. It is all too easy for the first test to be developed on the basis of its ability to reliably discriminate between candidates but having little to do with their clinical competence. The other danger is that the second hurdle, the clinical test, is not psychometrically sound.

Another approach is adaptive testing in which each component in the assessment is selected on the basis of performance on the previous component. The complexity of the strategy makes it practical only for computer-based tests of knowledge.

Sequential testing is a promising alternative and has been shown to be feasible but not very popular with candidates who may be distressed by being asked to undertake further testing.[7] It is based on the fact that a relatively short, and thus relatively unreliable test can quite accurately identify the candidates well above or well below the cut-off point. These candidates can safely be excused from further testing while the remainder are given a second round of the test. Consequently less resources are needed, with only those near the cutting score undertaking the full examination. Most organisations will not wish to become involved in such complex approaches or will have too few candidates to make it a major issue. For them, considerable efficiencies can be made by combining a written test with a relatively efficient clinical test such as an OSCE as long as both are developed from the same blueprint (see Case Study to follow).

Step 2: Decide on how the performance is to be recorded and captured
There are a number of technical issues to be addressed in scoring complex clinical assessments. Any organisation involved in using such procedures would be well advised to seek expert help in this matter. Issues to be addressed will include the design of scoring sheets; the training of simulated patients to score aspects of performance; and the training of examiners observing performance. A considerable literature exists on the relative merits of using checklists and rating scales. The current trend seems to be in favour of more global ratings, but we believe the best approach is one determined by the task being assessed. A skill with very clear component parts might best be scored on a detailed checklist while the assessment of effective patient communications might lend itself to a global scoring approach. Issues of systematic bias must be addressed using strategies such as multiple raters, large numbers of cases and, perhaps, training.

Step 3: Determine a method to score the cases or elements within cases
In this framework the term 'case' refers to a conceptual unit of the assessment. An example could be an item in a written examination or a station in an OSCE. Scores may be calculated as the sum of the points allocated to sub-components or as a percentage. Alternatively, they may be recorded as a simplified score (eg 0 – 1, pass/fail). The latter approach produces a less reproducible total score but such pass/fail-based scoring may be seen as more meaningful.

Having got the case score, the issue of how to combine them into a total score for decision-making purposes arises. The first approach will often lead to addition of case scores and then converting them to an overall percentile score. The second approach will lead to a decision-making system requiring a minimum number of stations to be passed. The more difficult issue comes when the final score must come (as it should come) from combining cases assessed using different test formats. Research in this area is limited.

Weighting of elements within a case is also something which must be considered even though it does not have a major effect on reproducibility of scores. We advocate that weighting should be part of the validation process, with more important elements being given greater weighting.

The use of scoring keys prepared before administration of the examination is a pre-requisite. The validity of the scoring keys is best checked by sufficient sampling of expert opinion and by pilot testing. The key should also be reviewed after the examination particularly if there is an intention to bank the item for repeat use.

Step 4: Take steps to avoid bias

While bias can affect written tests, it is a greater problem in clinical tests where observation and interaction between examiner and examinee are involved. The more difficult it is to define clearly the expected behaviour, and the more subjective the scoring, the greater the problem. Research in this area is slowly emerging but its impact on overall scores and pass/fail decisions is unclear. The best advice at present is to minimise the risk by reducing interaction between examiners and candidates to a minimum, objectifying marking schedules as far as is practical, training examiners and, most importantly, by observing a wide sample of performance using many examiners marking independently.

Step 5: Evaluate the need for equating scores across different examinations

Equating is the process of ensuring that scores on two different tests, developed from the same blueprint, are interchangeable. This process is necessary to ensure comparability of pass/fail decisions. The situation may arise when multiple forms of the same test are conducted at the same time but in different sites or when different tests are used at different times but are expected to be equivalent in content and standard.

Information is scarce on equating tests other than conventional written tests. The usual method of incorporating 'anchor' items used on previous tests is difficult to apply to clinical tests because of the limited number of 'items'. With large numbers of candidates, a broad-based equating based on normative statistics or standardisation of scores can be used.

Step 6: Ensure that trivialisation has not occurred

Trivialisation is a common but under-appreciated problem. It often applies to multiple-choice questions where isolated facts of no great merit may be included. Performance-based tests have been criticised for the same phenomenon. For example, checklists on OSCE stations may contain expected actions that are trivial. Avoidance of this problem simply requires care in ensuring that all elements being scored are relevant, important and appropriately weighted.

Setting standards for performance

Standard setting is the process of determining the score needed to pass an examination. It is clearly an issue of the greatest importance but one where the procedures used are often open to considerable criticism. It has to be appreciated that all standard setting procedures are, to a degree, arbitrary, but it is vital they are not capricious.

Two steps are involved in setting standards:

Step 1: Determine the type of standard desired and an appropriate method of standard setting

Standards are classified as relative or absolute. Relative standards are the most commonly used and are statistically based. For example, the bottom 10% fail or any student scoring less than one standard deviation below the mean fails. Such an approach is not generally regarded as conceptually appropriate for tests of clinical competence.

Absolute standards are based on an analysis of the content of the examination and the setting of a score that must be achieved to pass. Unfortunately the methods of doing this have been developed primarily for written tests and are cumbersome. Examples of such procedures are the Angoff, Ebel and Hofstee methods. All require decisions to be taken by experts on an estimate of the expected item scores of a borderline candidate. Modification of these procedures is being actively investigated for use in clinical examinations, an example being one developed by the Medical Council of Canada.[8]

An alternative approach is to use a reference group. This method entails putting a large sample of candidates who are expected to be at or above the standard through the test and use their performance data to generate a minimum standard. The practicalities of this preclude its use in most cases, but an example is provided by the new General Medical Council Performance Procedures. In the general practice competence test component, the standard of the written test is determined by having the test undertaken by a large sample of UK general practitioners.

Step 2: Develop procedures for communicating the results

Regardless of how scores are formed and standards set, all reported scores must be reliable and valid. Sub-scores should not be reported unless they reach acceptable levels of reliability. Unfortunately this is often not the case in clinical examinations where pass/fail decisions may be based on unreliable data such as a single long-case assessment.

It is highly desirable that information about all assessment procedures and decision-making processes is totally transparent. A clear written document should be available to all candidates.

SUMMARY

The basis of developing a good test of clinical competence is careful and thorough planning using current best evidence-based assessment practice. Personal opinion and approaches simply based on tradition are no longer justifiable. Research over the last 20 years has advanced enormously our ability to deliver high quality clinical assessment. While more research is required, there can be no excuse for any organisation to continue with outmoded practice with unacceptable levels of reliability and validity.

CASE STUDIES

Three case studies reflecting the personal experience of the authors will be described. They will help by illustrating how the guidelines described above have been put into practice. The first relates to a final year undergraduate examination, the second to the development of a national certification examination and the third to the revalidation of the performance of established clinicians.

One: Developing a multi-station assessment of competence

In places like the UK and Australia there are no national licensing examinations at the undergraduate level. Medical schools are accredited by national Medical Councils which approve their curricula-including assessment procedures. The university medical degree is accepted as a sufficient credential for provisional registration to practice as a junior doctor under supervision. Critical evaluation of procedures in use in medical schools has revealed that many have relied on the traditional clinical examination which has proven limitations in content validity and reliability. This case study will describe the ongoing development of a multi-disciplinary final year examination first introduced at the University of Adelaide in 1979.[9]

This examination has been constructed according to a blueprint based on the competencies required of an intern (PRHO). The content validity was established by identifying the problems an intern would have to deal with during their work on the wards or in the emergency department and was identified by consensus. The competencies were obtaining the database, clinical assessment/diagnostic acumen, tests and procedures, treatment and implementing care.[10]

It became clear that assessing competence using this approach did not fit logically into the conventional disciplinary-based final year examination. Initially, it became an integrated assessment conducted by the departments of medicine and surgery. Subsequently other departments became involved. A review of test methodology also made it clear that that the traditional clinical examination was too unreliable for such an important assessment. It was decided to introduce an OSCE together with a free-response short-answer paper.

In 1988 we were able to report some psychometric analyses of this approach which identified several practical and logistic problems.[11] For example, we showed that an examination based on an OSCE alone would have to be prohibitively long (about six hours) to obtain scores that were reliable enough for high stakes decision-making. However, we were also able to demonstrate that our strategy of appropriately combining written and OSCE components reduced the required testing time to more manageable proportions without compromising validity.

By the mid-1990s, the examination had achieved stability with a high level of support and acceptance by students and the institution. The clinical component now consisted of a 15-station OSCE lasting 90 minutes. This comprised nine stations involving interactions with patients (real and simulated) and four static stations involving interpretation of clinical data (eg X-rays, clinical photos). The written component lasts 120 minutes and has two sections. The first contains 75 free response questions and the second the equivalent of another six static stations (eg interpretation of ECGs and laboratory data).

Psychometric analyses in the 1980s showed the reliability of the overall test to be 0.73 significantly short of the minimally accepted standard for high stakes tests of 0.80. The reliabilities of the components were, of course, much less, with the OSCE being of the order of 0.5 and the written test being approximately 0.7. The analysis of the 1996 data showed a considerable improvement, with the equivalent figures being 0.81, 0.65 and 0.8.[12] The overall quality had now achieved a level that would be defensible if legally challenged, both on validity and reliability grounds, an important consideration in an age of increasing litigation.

This case study demonstrates the value of an organised approach to test development bases on sound principles of educational measurement.

Two: Establishing content validity for the PLAB test

In 1998 the GMC initiated a wide-ranging and fundamental review of the Professional and Linguistic Assessments Board (PLAB) test. The test dates from 1974 and was originally established to assess the knowledge, skills and linguistic ability of applicants for temporary (now limited) registration. In 1999 the test is a high stakes examination which assesses the competence of doctors who qualify outside the UK and European Economic Area and who wish to gain limited registration. The Council has determined that the standard of the test will be the standard expected of doctors about to commence their first SHO post. The emphasis of the test will be on common and important conditions seen by SHOs and the generic management of life-threatening situations, with an emphasis on clinical management and science as applied to clinical problems.

This case study will describe the way the Sub-group on the Standard and Scope of the Test and the Testing Method has approached the task of constructing a content blueprint for the examination and selecting test methods for the future. It can be seen as an established procedure under continuing development.

With the purpose of the test clearly defined, the first step in constructing the overall blueprint was to establish the problems and tasks that SHOs starting their first job could reasonably be expected to meet and undertake. Several databases were consulted:

■ a survey of SHOs who had passed the PLAB test to establish what problems they had to deal with in practice;
■ a survey of A&E consultants to discover their views on essential knowledge and skills for SHOs in their first job;
■ a review of admissions to a district general hospital (DGH) via A&E over a six-month period;
■ a survey of consecutive attendances at two DGHs over 48 hours;
■ a list of common and non-rare important problems and more common cancers presenting in general practice based on the OPCS Morbidity Statistics from General Practice; and
■ core cases from the Liverpool and Manchester undergraduate curricula.[13]

The most common and important problems were derived by taking all of those mentioned by at least 40% of the respondents in the surveys, the top five conditions by diagnosis or by presentation from the DGH and admission data and all of the consecutive attendances at A&E. The most common and important GP problems were selected by LS and all of the undergraduate core cases were included. The problems were classified into body systems, with an additional section for paediatrics. As an example, the entries for psychiatry are shown in Figure 2. After inspecting these entries, the sub-group members selected conditions as diagnoses, presenting problems or practical skills for inclusion in the final blueprint. The selections for psychiatry were alcohol and drug abuse, anxiety, assessing suicide risk, assessment of mental state, dealing with aggression, grief and anger, dementia, depression, overdoses/other self harm and psychoses (principally schizophrenia). These became one arm of the blueprint.

The other dimension for the overall blueprint was derived from *Good Medical Practice*, the GMC guidance to all doctors on the Register, and the recent publication on the PRHO year, *The New Doctor.* Generic attributes to be expected of all SHOs were used to form a matrix with the problems/presentations and practical skills selected in the manner described above. A section of the final blueprint is shown in Figure 3. The problems are listed in alphabetical order, as the test will be case based rather than discipline or systems based.

The final step in devising the blueprint was to select problems and attributes that will be over-sampled, based on their incidence and/or their danger to life, and conditions (eg asthma) for which paediatric questions must be written. The sub-group made decisions about which attributes are most important, for SHOs, for example, diagnosis and prescribing will be over-sampled. For some conditions the ability to recognise and make initial decisions will be all that is required, for others, management and follow-up will be expected. Individual tests will be drawn up from the item banks according to these rules and the performance of items in previous diets.

This blueprint is for the entire test, and will be used to draw the content for both the written test and the OSCE. Some items naturally lend themselves to a particular method, for example bladder catheterisation will be assessed in the OSCE using a manikin. After considering test methods, several attributes expected of SHOs are not suitable for testing in an examination and will be delegated to formal appraisal during the period of limited registration. These are: teamwork; access to medical records/data protection; peer review; use of resources; and using information storage and retrieval systems appropriately.

Figure 2. Developing the PLAB blueprint: common and important problems in psychiatry according to different data sources

DATA SOURCE	SIEO/COMMON >40 PERCENT OF RESPONDENTS	DGH CASE MIX/ADMISSIONS VIA A&E/COMMON SUMMER SIX MONTHS	DGH SNAPSHOT OF A/E ATTENDANCES IN 42 HOURS IN JULY	CONSULTANTS CONSENSUS ON IMPORTANT PROBLEMS >40 PERCENT RESPONDENTS	COMMON AND RARE IMPORTANT PROBLEMS AND COMMONEST CANCERS PRESENTING IN GENERAL PRACTICE OPCS MORBIDITY STATISTICS	CASES FROM THE PROBLEMS BASED CURRICULUM AT LIVERPOOL additional cases from Manchester core curriculum
by diagnosis	Dementia Depression		Depression Psychosis	Depression Psychosis Toxic confusional state	Anxiety Dementia Depression Schizophrenia	Anorexia nervosa Anxiety Chronic fatigue syndrome Dementia Depression Mania Parasuicide Phobias Post traumatic stress Schizophrenia
by problem	Alcohol and drug abuse Depression	Alcohol and drug abuse Overdoses	Deliberate self harm Hyperventilation Overdoses	Alcohol and drug abuse	Alcohol and drug abuse	Alcohol and drug abuse Aggression/violence Panic attack Sleep disturbances Somatisation
by practical	Assess mental state Deal with aggression/grief/anger			Assess mental state Deal with aggression/grief/anger Assess suicide risk		

Figure 3. A section of the final PLAB blueprint

Problems, diagnosis and practical skills listed in alphabetical order form a matrix with examples of attributes expected of all SHOs.

Definition of the clinical tasks within each cell, the level of resolution expected from an SHO, the selection of test method and preparation of relevant test items must follow.

	Decision making	Management plan	Prescribing including writing a prescription and calculating a drug dose	Listening, explaining, involving patients in decisions	Dealing with complaints
Bruising bleeding purpura					
Burns					
Cataract					
Cervical cancer					
Cervical smear					
Chest pain[1]					

[1] Chest pain is both common and important and will be over sampled

The revised PLAB test will be relevant to practice in the UK, support SHOs in their first appointments, and should improve quality of care. This must be established through research. When the blueprint is completed it will be made available to candidates who for the first time will have a syllabus to prepare for. The test will have content validity, which is necessary but not sufficient for a test of the highest quality. The other aspects described in our introductory section are also being reviewed and implemented.

Three: Peer review of performance of established clinicians

Since changes to the *Medical Act* in 1997, the GMC has undertaken one of the most difficult tasks of all – assessing the competence and performance of doctors on the Register about whom sufficient concerns have been raised for a referral to be made to the GMC's *Fitness to Practice* procedures. This case study will describe how the guidelines were used to develop its procedures from the conceptual stages through to their implementation in practice with particular emphasis on peer review.

The purpose of the assessments of performance within the performance procedures was determined by the GMC, and the task of the assessors is to identify and document deficient performance sufficiently serious to call the doctor's registration into question. Complete information about the procedures is available from the GMC.

The assessments have been developed and piloted by 20 working groups which together have provided coverage for the entire profession. The group members recognised the complex relationship that exists between performance (does do) and competence (can do). The decision was taken early to assess performance in practice first followed by tests of competence if serious deficiency cannot confidently be ruled out during peer review. Assessments of performance and competence are different and pose different challenges in relation to reliability and validity. This case study describes the performance-based aspects.

The validity of the overall review process derives from the attributes expected of any registered doctor as set out in *Good Medical Practice* and the content of the clinical practice of the doctor being reviewed. They form the two dimensions of the overall blueprint for both phases of the assessment. The methods have been chosen and developed to enable assessment of each area during peer review at the place of practice.[14]

The peer review visit is conducted by two medical and one lay assessor over two full days. While they are to some extent customised to individual disciplines, all doctors entering the *Performance Procedures* complete an extended CV in order to present their education, training, experience, and actual clinical practice including audit data. All practitioners will normally encounter assessment of medical record-keeping, discussion of cases based on their own records (case-based oral) observation of consultations and interviews with third parties. There will also be introductory and final structured interviews with the full assessment team and a site tour to determine the context of practice. All of the assessments are structured in a similar way with the judgements of assessors being recorded against a uniform set of criteria. The report to the GMC is written using a template common to the entire profession based on headings that derive from *Good Medical Practice.* The conclusions of the assessors must be supported by documented evidence from multiple sources.

An example of part of the instrument for assessing medical record-keeping for surgeons is shown in Figure 4. At least 50 records are inspected. Other parts of the instrument look at out-patient and in-patient record-keeping, fully aware that notes are often made by juniors, and that one doctor rarely takes responsibility for the care of the patient from referral to discharge from follow-up. The criteria were developed by surgeons in active practice and piloted during validation visits. The assessors apply the standard they embody as peers.

One of the foundation principles of the GMC performance assessments is the role of the assessors as peers of the doctor. The training of assessors is of great importance in developing peer review for this very high stakes assessment. They must understand and be confident in their role, and be given the right tools to carry it out. Their tasks are summarised in Figure 5. One of the successes of the program has been the involvement of lay assessors in every aspect of development and implementation of the assessments. Medical and lay assessors have trained together and several teams have carried out assessments that have now stood legal challenge.

CONCLUSIONS: IMPLICATIONS FOR SURGERY

The assessment of surgeons, whether established or in training, is a focus of public concern. Few other activities in medicine have their potential for good or harm so generally discussed. Overall, the development of a blueprint and the selection of methods for assessment of competence and performance is the same as for other disciplines. But while many practitioners consider that the most important aspect of the discipline is accurate diagnosis and excellent decision-making (the right operation at the right time), there is a growing interest in the assessment of practical skills. Although outcome measures can give a measure of the performance of teams, there is further work to do in developing the assessment of an individual surgeon's practical ability. During training, at the early stages, basic skills can be assessed in a skills laboratory. Individuals who are unsuited to the discipline because of very poor manual dexterity should be identified at this stage and counselled. Assessment of entire procedures is much more difficult as experienced individuals have different ways of achieving excellent outcomes. It will be necessary to develop assessments

Figure 4. Criteria for assessing surgical record keeping used by assessors in the GMC performance procedures

CRITERIA		ACCEPTABLE	CAUSE FOR CONCERN	UNACCEPTABLE
OPERATION NOTES	PRESENT & DATED	Consented operation note is dated and signed in notes and operation book in theatre.	Date only recorded. Consent not recorded. Theatre book not filled in.	No entry by surgeons. All information contained in the anaesthetic notes.
	WHAT WAS DONE & WHO BY	Incision Operation Closure Drains Surgeon	Information complete and could possibly cause a problem for another surgeon following up.	Impossible to discover what done from the operation notes. Identity of the surgeon unclear.
	HOW IT WAS DONE	It is possible to discover which surgical techniques were employed. Good diagrams.	Illegible, parts difficult to follow. The description relies on the imagination of the reader to complete it.	Wholly illegible or missing.
	ANY PROBLEMS DURING THE PROCEDURE	Documentation of: - bleeding - inadvertent damage to other structures - unplanned procedures - other colleagues called to help. Patient informed.	Problems incompletely documented. Surgeon left theatre aware problem not corrected.	Attempts to conceal mistakes. Failure to resolve situation. Failure to acknowledge problem.
	POST OPERATIVE INSTRUCTIONS	Clear instructions about: - post-op analgesia - fluids, drains, catheters and sutures. Reasons will documented, in notes, letters and nursing notes.	Incomplete post-op instructions. Other staff called to clarify. Failure to visit post operatively.	No follow up after pleas by patient/GP on surgical staff. Failure to return to hospital/theatre when evidence strongly in favour of doing so.
	DID THE PATIENT RETURN TO THEATRE	Clear details why and names or surgeons involved. Planned/unplanned Complications, consent	Dates only recorded. Details scant or unclear.	No notes or evasive. Died/significant morbidity due to delay in decision.

Figure 5. The tasks of assessors undertaking peer review of performance in practice

- To gather evidence
- To judge the evidence against criteria
- To apply a standard which they embody as peers but which is supported by valid criteria and evidence based standards where they exist
- To report their findings in a way that provides feedback and withstands challenge

Before conducting peer review
- understanding of the principles of assessment
- the difference between tests of competence and assessment of performance
- planning a visit and reviewing the documentation
- gaining familiarity with the criteria and standards and how they are recorded
- triangulation of evidence

During a visit
- the conduct of a visit (eg: level of formality)
- rigour and structure combined with warmth and encouragement
- completing the docmentation
- working as a team member
- decision making and report writing
- giving feedback, including bad news

based on peer review which include informed scrutiny of audit data and direct observation of practical procedures. For most practitioners the opportunity to observe a colleague working is a treat, and the debate and learning that it engenders is immensely valuable. If peer review can be developed with this in mind, with reviewers trained to give feedback in a constructive way, the benefits will be tangible.

Finally, the systematic construction of an assessment blueprint for surgeons will ultimately be based on *Good Medical Practice.* Communication and relationships with patients must be a part of it. Basic communication skills are tested in the MRCS examination. The government user and patient survey, which will be introduced as part of clinical governance, will also provide data. Local peer review between surgical teams could provide an opportunity to involve trained lay assessors, who will be able to observe consultations and give feedback. Most surgeons are excellent communicators; introduction of this aspect into assessment will finally give the lie to the stereotype that says otherwise.

References

1.   Southgate L, Dauphinee D. Maintaining standards in British and Canadian medicine: the developing role of the regulatory bodies. *BMJ* 1998: 316;697-700.

2.   Newble D (editor), Guidelines for the development of effective and efficient procedures for the assessment of clinical competence. In: Newble D, Jolly B, Wakeford R, editors. *The Certification and Recertification of Doctors: Issues in the Assessment of Clinical Competence.* Cambridge: Cambridge University Press; 1994. p69-91.

3.   Newble D, Dawson B (eds), Dauphinee D, Macdonald M, Mulholland H, Page G, Swanson D, Thomson A. Guidelines for assessing clinical competence. *Teaching and Learning in Medicine* 1994:6:213-220.

4.   Van der Vleuten C, Newble D (editors) Methods of assessing in certification. In Newble D, Jolly B, Wakeford R, editors. *The Certification and Recertification of Doctors: Issues in the Assessment of Clinical Competence.* Cambridge: Cambridge University Press; 1994; p105-125.

5.   Clyman SG, Melnick DE, Clauser BE. Computer-based case simulations. In Mansell EL, Bashook PG, editors. *Assessing Clinical Reasoning: The Oral Examination and Alternative Methods.* Chicago, Illinois: American Board of Medical Specialties; 1995. p. 139-149.

6.   Rothman AI, Blackmore DE, Dauphinee WD, Reznick R. Test of sequential testing in two years results of Part 2 of the Medical Council of Canada Qualifying Examination. *Acad. Med.* 1997; 72(supp10):522-524.

7.   Dauphinee WD, Blackmore DE, Smee SM, Rothman AI, Desmarchais J, Reznick RJ. Adaptive testing: a report on the results and myths arising from uthe use of a sequences OSCE for national licensure. *Proceedings of the 8th International Ottawa Conference on Medical Education and Assessment;* 1998 July 12-15; Philadelphia, USA (in press).

8.   Dauphinee WD, Blackmore DE, Smee SM, Rothman AI, Reznick R. Using the judgements of physician examiners in setting the standards for a national multicentre high stakes OSCE. *Advances in Health Science Education* 1997; 2:201-211.

9.   Newble DI, Elmslie RG. A new approach to the final examinations in Medicine and Surgery. *Lancet* 1981:517-518.

10.   Newble DI, Hoare J, Elmslie RG. The validity and reliability of a new examination of the clinical competence of medical students. *Med Educ* 1981; 15:46-52.

11.   Newble DI, Swanson DB. Psychometric characteristics of the objective structured clinical examination. *Med. Educ.* 1988; 22:325-334.

12.   Newble DI, Swanson DB. Improving the quality of a multi-disciplinary test of clinical competence: a longitudinal study. *Proceedings of the 8th International Ottawa Conference on Medical Education and Assessment;* 1998 July 12-15; Philadelphia, USA (in press).

13.   O'Neill P, Metcalfe D, David T. The core content of the undergraduate curriculum in Manchester. *Med Educ* 1999; 33:121-129.

14.   Southgate L, Ayres B, Elkington A, Hatch D, Johnson N, Jolly B, Mulholland H, Tombleson P. Blueprint *The Poorly performing doctor in the UK: the development and implementation of a comprehensive for assessment by the General Medical Council.*

15.   NHS Executive. *The New NHS, Modern and Dependable: a National Framework for Assessing Performance.* London: Department of Health, 1998.

Objectifying Skills Assessment: Bench Model Solutions

Deepak Dath, MD, FRCSC

Education Research Fellow at the University of Toronto

Richard K Reznick, MD, Med., FRCSC, FACS

Professor of Surgery at University of Toronto
Director, University of Toronto, Faculty of Medicine, Centre for Research in
Education at University Health Network

Abstract

Surgeons need to be quite technically adept. A rigorous training apprenticeship usually ensures that surgeons' technical skill is high but the assessment of such skill in the training programs is generally subjective. A more objective method of technical skill assessment would help to justify promotion of trainees through their programs and ensure that certifying bodies grant credentials appropriately. Objective evaluation of technical skill is also useful in providing feedback during training.

Ethical issues and the subjective nature of the operating environment encourage the development of technical assessment platforms outside the operating room. Although cadaver and live animal models show greater operative fidelity, their disadvantages include availability, expense and ethical issues of use. Bench models offer a standardised environment with variable face validity and lower cost. An objective structured assessment of technical skill (OSATS) examination format has been developed and tested using such bench models. Candidates are required to rotate from station to station performing defined tasks while being evaluated by trained surgeons using a standardised checklist and a global rating scale. The examination shows high reliability and construct validity and is suitable for certification decisions. OSATS examinations are expensive and require significant expertise in their administration. The developers have shown that the examination can be administered peripherally from a central site with maintenance of its psychometric properties. The OSATS format ensures that newer technologies such as virtual reality computer simulations can be incorporated as they become available.

INTRODUCTION

Deftness is an attribute that is colloquially credited to all surgeons. The phrase 'the hands of a surgeon' is used to describe someone who possesses exceptional manual dexterity. Surgeons are simply expected to possess exceptional technical skill because a patient could potentially pay a high price for a surgeon's technical ineptitude. However, surgeons themselves do not reduce their primary qualities and strengths to their technical skill. Spencer[1] stated that 'a skilfully performed task comprises 75% decision-making and 25% manual dexterity', de-emphasising the relative importance of technical skills in the training of surgeons. Because the 25% of surgery that comprises technical skill is crucial to the practice of the profession, Barnes[2] proposed that the surgical education community has a responsibility to pay attention to the way that surgical skills are taught and assessed. In fact, this 25% is likely the largest individual component of a surgeon's expertise and one not readily assumed by other specialists. It is therefore vital to optimise technical training and to ensure that the graduates of surgical training programmes have acquired a high level of technical expertise.

Surgical skill has always been taught with the pupil at the master's elbow. Historically, the French, English and German systems of training physicians used this mentored, apprenticeship approach. Halstead, who trained in Europe, is credited with introducing and establishing the technique of a mentored apprenticeship of graded responsibility and experience[3] to surgical training programs in North America at the turn of the century. Since that time, surgical trainees have been continually subjectively assessed by their mentors and are expected to have achieved intellectual and technical competence if they progressed to the end of their training. Most often, a professional board then certifies trainees as surgeons on passing written and oral exams. There is usually no formal assessment of skill, although technical competence has always been an important part of the promotion of a resident through a training program.

RATIONALE FOR TECHNICAL SKILLS ASSESSMENT

There are three main categories of assessment regarding any aspect of performance during surgical training. These include formative evaluation, summative evaluation, and evaluation of continued competence. The assessment methods for each of these purposes may be different. Formative assessment implies an ongoing method of providing feedback to the trainees. This can be relatively informal, such as a preceptor providing interim reports to a resident regarding technical performance. Alternatively it can be more formal, with every operation being subject to a specific method of assessment. Kopta[4] stated that the reduction of technical evaluation into specific components allows for the concrete assessment of technical performance.

Summative evaluation implies arriving at a final decision or grade for a particular aspect of performance. This usually takes the form of a discrete examination which is used as a final assessment method to make decisions about progress through training or for certification and/or licensure.

Assessment also plays a vital role in assuring the maintenance of competence. Currently, licensure is granted upon an assessment at the end of formal training that may or may not include an element of technical skill evaluation. There is an urge to progress toward regular mandatory assessment of competence, but currently, in most countries, this does not include technical skill assessment. Issues surrounding the regular assessment of technical skills abound and include feasibility, validity and reliability of such testing. However, the public perception of accountability extends to include medical care, so issues that currently seem to be barriers will have to be resolved so that assessment of continued technical competence becomes a reality. Assessment of technical competence would probably be simplified to an initial assessment at licensure with ongoing assessments of technical skill only for surgeons training in new procedures. Surgical outcome audits might be the method used to identify individuals who need to have their technical competence reassessed.

Residency programs currently use a number of different types of assessment tools and criteria to judge the progress of their residents through a program. Such tools include in-training evaluations, oral examinations and written examinations. From these evaluations, it is expected that trainees will be assessed in the many dimensions of surgical competence, some directly observed and some inferred. These examinations have done a good job in assessing surgical knowledge and surgical judgement but have not succeeded in formally assessing technical skill. To be sure, surgeons have taken seriously their mandate to attest the surgical competence of their trainees through informal evaluation in the operating room. However, in most instances, this type of assessment has been unstructured and lacks the fundamental psychometric properties of a successful evaluation system.

Analysing surgical skill training and developing good methods of assessment have proved to be difficult tasks. Yet, without good methods of assessment, no objective statements can be made about the technical ability of graduating surgeons and no serious effort put in to improve technical training and skills. Surgical skills, therefore, need to be assessed in residency programs. However, the need to assess surgical skills only partly rests with residency programs. Certifying bodies must also improve their ability to assess technical skill and continuing education programs that teach new skills or offer upgrading of skills will need to include components that verify the acquisition of these skills in their participants.

There is a growing atmosphere of public expectation that the medical profession improve its ability to ensure the competence of its members. This expectation has legal implications in the case of unnecessarily poor patient outcomes (surgical misadventure). The usual venue for skills training and assessment is the operating room and the usual method is a global assessment of competence by the staff surgeon supervising the resident. However, economic considerations preclude the use of more operating room time for educational activity. The ethical basis of using the operating room for training and assessment has also been questioned. Training and assessment must be transferred to another venue that is less expensive and therefore more accessible. In the effort to improve training programs in surgery, program changes will inevitably occur. First, however, programs must assess the skill of their residents before implementing any changes to their training program to determine the current standard that they achieve. Skill assessment after implementation of a change in the program will then help to determine whether that change is beneficial. How can technical skill assessment be implemented in the most objective way to satisfy the many needs that have been outlined?

In this chapter, we will outline the current methods available to assess technical skill. In addition, we will highlight the development of a new method of assessing technical skill, the Objective Structured Assessment of Technical Skill (OSATS). In so doing, we will comment on the strengths and weaknesses of different assessment formats and speculate on the utility of newer methods that may be available in the future.

MODELS USED TO TEST SURGICAL SKILLS

Patients

The ethical validity of teaching technical skills on patients in the operating room has been questioned for some time. Patients will sometimes ask their surgeons whether the surgeons themselves will be performing the operation. Inevitably, some mention is made of the fact that residents assist in the operation, although the residents might in fact be expected to perform the bulk of the operation. However, the ethical issues surrounding the degree of a resident's participation in a particular patient's operation are not uniformly delineated. It would be difficult to regularly obtain consent from patients to have residents be assessed for technical skill during their surgeries, since the testing of competence implies the possibility of a lack of expertise.

However, operating on patients represents the real world experience that residents will be expected to face at the completion of their training. There can be no more valid test than in such a real situation. This realism does pose a problem in the objectivity of assessment since it limits standardisation. Realism and standardisation are mutually discrepant objectives in the testing of surgical skills. It is difficult to standardise surgical procedures, to standardise the resident's level of participation in the case and to standardise the frame of reference as to the level of expectation for performance by different levels of trainees. How, for instance, would a junior resident be evaluated in the performance of a laparoscopic cholecystectomy if the supervising surgeon assumed control early in the case? Similarly, it would be impossible to discriminate between the competencies of senior residents who performed uncomplicated procedures that did not adequately challenge their abilities or residents at the same level of training who were assessed on more difficult cases. If regular assessment of technical competence is to succeed, evaluation in other environments that can be standardised must complement the evaluations that take place in the operating room.

Cadavers

Cadavers have the same anatomic relations as patients. They are expensive for use in testing since only a limited number of procedures can be assessed per cadaver and because they are not reusable. Cadavers also may not be suitable for some procedures such as laparoscopic surgery. The feel of the tissues is different and there is no bleeding to control during dissection. There is variability in availability of cadavers and cadavers may present unexpected variability of anatomy. Previous operations and the resulting scar tissue may complicate procedures on cadavers. Cadavers too, are inappropriate for use in regular skills evaluation.

Animal models

Live animals are a common platform for the teaching and assessment of surgical procedures. Live animals are accessible and have many advantages such as tactile validity and the realism of living, breathing and bleeding tissue. However, there are several disadvantages to the use of animals. Firstly, are the ethical issues which have constrained the use of animal altogether in some jurisdictions. Secondly, animals are expensive and require specialised facilities. Thirdly, anatomic relations may be sufficiently different from humans to minimise the degree of transfer of learned skill from an animal to the human reality.

Stotter and colleagues[5] developed lyophylised, freeze-dried animal tissue for bench training of surgical skills in 1986 and the Anastomosis Workshop at The Royal College of Surgeons in England had been using bench models that incorporate animal tissue for some time before that.[6] With jigs from the workshop to hold the animal specimen, reasonably good representation of tissue substrate was made available for practising technical skills. This bench model of animal tissue merits further investigation as an instrument for skill assessment.

Synthetic models

Low fidelity models are inexpensive and sometimes reusable depending on the simulation being attempted. Face validity is the biggest drawback to their use since some models may not represent the anatomy well in their geometry or tactile properties. These may be of greater use for general practice prior to testing and for the testing of junior trainees where the operator's familiarity with instruments and the operating environment might be of primary interest.

High fidelity models are more expensive and less likely to be reusable. Face validity may be quite good for some models. Materials have been developed to represent the structural qualities of blood vessels and organic tissues. Certain companies have succeeded in using these materials to simulate the geometry of the anatomy well. Plastic models are quite portable and do not potentially transmit diseases as patients, cadavers and animal models might. The greatest drawback of the plastic models is still their limited reaction to manipulation – the tissue does not slip, bend or cut, nor is it sewed up like organic tissue and it does not bleed. The degree of transfer of learned skills from non-human models to the human reality is largely unknown.

The future for computer-based surgical simulations is bright. As software and hardware continues on their exponential curves of development, we can expect the introduction of virtual reality models of surgical operations that closely simulate the real world. At present, however, the use of computer simulations to teach and test surgical skill is limited.

MODELS OF SKILL ASSESSMENT

Procedural lists

This is a widely used technique for assessing skills. Most programs suggest or require that their residents keep surgical logs. Residents record each procedure according to their level of participation. Some credential-bestowing organisations rely on the number of procedures performed as adjuncts to attestations from program directors that residents are competent in the technical aspects of surgery.

The procedural tallies also ensure experience over a defined range of operations. This process relies on the assumption that residency training programs would oversee the day-to-day technical ability of candidates and ensure that enough practice and training were had to assure their technical competence before advancing them to the examination. This is not an unreasonable assumption to be made. Surgical programs consider the matter of technical skill to be an important issue and have always striven to ensure the technical competence of their residents.

The procedure list is a crude surrogate for the assessment of technical skill. Its only redeeming quality is its ability to assure the depth and breadth of a resident's operative experience. No conclusions can be drawn as to the level of technical expertise that any candidate achieves. The assessment of technical competence in this method truly rests with the candidate's residency supervisors who can determine whether the candidate's technical skill deserves graduation from the program. Technical competence, therefore, can vary widely from program to program.

In-training evaluations

The technical component of surgical in-training evaluations usually consists of global assessments rendered on a rating form. These forms are completed at the end of a rotation, reflecting the overall impression of the supervisors on particular dimensions as based on their recall of the resident's performance over the length of the rotation. Clearly, such an exit evaluation may be overly subjective.

Other problems with the current system of global rating scales stem from the manner of their administration. Rating surgeons rarely receive any form of 'rater' training, there is often tremendous variation in the stringency and leniency of raters and residents are often assessed by only one rater.

These factors have resulted in the lack of reliability of this assessment approach which lessens the confidence with which one can interpret the results. To be sure, it is vital to assess performance displayed during the training years. It is real world performance in real situations, free of biases that occur during discrete examination periods. The challenge remains to develop a comprehensive system of assessing the day-to-day technical activities of the residents that is objective and which can reward the resident with feedback.

Direct observation in the operating room with criteria

One method of avoiding the subjectivity of the general global assessment in the operating room is to have surgeons observe residents' performances and rate them using highly structured checklists. These checklists outline the steps necessary to complete a procedure and can be very objective. For example, Winckel and colleagues[7] developed a structured technical skills assessment form (STSAF) to help evaluate technical skills in the operating room. The STSAF is a highly structured checklist consisting of an average of 120 items that allows surgeons to observe residents' operative performance on a particular operation and rate them objectively on each of the checklist components. The STSAF also includes an expanded summary scale in a global rating format to capture the assessment of the concepts of technical competence, focusing on surgical behaviours instead of surgical manoeuvres. The global rating rating form looks at a different dimension of performance and assesses a complex amalgam of surgical issues rather than focusing strictly on the task.

Winckel and colleagues constructed STSAFs for open cholecystectomies, open hernia repairs and bowel resections, evaluating 12 residents over 41 operations with 26 operations being evaluated by two raters. Inter-rater reliability was 0.78 and 0.73 for the checklists and global rating scales, with the two instruments being highly correlated (Pearson correlation coefficient = 0.89). The checklist scores also discriminated effectively between junior and senior trainees, implying construct validity.

The checklist approach in an operative setting is ideal for providing specific feedback on the technical skill of residents. It can be used whenever the supervising surgeon feels that such feedback would be beneficial to the resident. Its drawback is that it requires the presence of an expert observer throughout the operation although the surgeon assisting the resident can complete a global assessment at the end of the operation. The global assessment takes less time to complete so it can easily be done several times for each resident on each rotation. This would help to provide a sound evaluation of the resident's technical performance on a rotation.

OSATS

The Surgical Education Group at the University of Toronto has developed a bench model examination for surgical skills called the Objective Structured Assessment of Technical Skills (OSATS). [8-11] This examination uses bench model simulations of surgical tasks to assess performance. Elements of simulated operations are selected for evaluation rather than the whole procedure itself. Residents rotate from task to task performing technical skills while being observed by trained surgeons. This examination is modelled after the Objective Structured Clinical Examination (OSCE) which has been used for the past two decades to assess clinical skills such as taking a history, doing a physical examination, or communicating with patients. The OSCE technology has been adapted for the assessment of technical skills.

The specific parts of an operation that are to be tested are gleaned from the objectives of training of the residency program. Once a topic is chosen, content experts then generate checklists that are used in the evaluation process. Each testing unit or 'station' is checked and refined as part of an elaborate validation process.

The typical exam involves residents rotating on through eight 15-minute stations. While performing elements of a technical task, they are observed and rated by qualified surgeons who mark from two scoring schemes. The first is a task-specific checklist, a scoring rubric that delineates whether a resident has or has not performed a particular element of the procedure (Figure 1). The second is a global rating scale which looks at surgical behaviours (Figure 2). Since its development, there have been several iterations of the OSATS and it is now administered on a yearly basis as part of the training program at the University of Toronto. The Surgical Education Group has conducted several studies in an attempt to further refine the examination, assess its reliability, and analyse its validity.

An initial study by Martin and colleagues[8] compared live animals to bench models. It was felt, at that time, that live animal simulations represented the gold standard to which bench model simulations would have to compare. This study showed that the OSATS was a feasible model for testing technical skills. It showed that the bench model and live models were equally effective in discriminating between different levels of trainees. This was true for scores in general and also true for a specific station. Therefore, if a resident had performed well on a bowel anastamosis in a pig, that resident was likely to perform well on a bowel anastamosis using a bench model simulation.

Figure 1.   Sample OSATS checklist

Small Bowel Anastamosis

INSTRUCTIONS TO CANDIDATES

You have just resected a segment of small bowel. Perform a single layer, interrupted, end to end anastamosis to restore continuity.

ITEM	Not Done or Incorrect	Done Correctly
1. Bowel oriented mesenteric border to mesenteric border, no twisting	0	1
2. Stay sutures held with snaps	0	1
3. Selects appropriate needle driver (Gen surg, medtip/med or short length)	0	1
4. Selects appropriate suture (atraumatic, 3.0/4.0, PDS/Dexon/Vicryl/silk)	0	1
5. Needle loaded 1/2 to 2/3 from tip	0	1
6. Index used to stabilize needle driver	0	1
7. Needle enters bowel at right angles 80% of bites	0	1
8. Single attempt at needle passage through bowel 90% of bites	0	1
9. Follow through on curve of needle on entrance on 80% of bites	0	1
10. Follow through on curve of needle on exit on 80% of bites	0	1
11. Forceps used on seromuscular layer of bowel only majority of time	0	1
12. Minimal damage with forceps	0	1
13. Uses forceps to handle needle	0	1
14. Inverting sutures	0	1
15. Suture spacing 3 to 5 mm	0	1
16. Equal bites on each side 80% of bites	0	1
17. Individual bites each side 90% of bites	0	1
18. Square knots	0	1
19. Minimum three throws on knots	0	1
20. Suture cut to appropriate length (does not interfere with next stitch)	0	1
21. No mucosal pouting	0	1
22. Apposition of bowel without excessive tension on sutures.	0	1
MAXIMUM TOTAL SCORE		**(22)**
TOTAL SCORE		

Figure 2. Sample global rating scale

GLOBAL RATING SCALE OF OPERATIVE PERFORMANCE

Please circle the number corresponding to the candidate's performance, **regardless of the candidates level of training.**

Respect for tissue

1	2	3	4	5
Frequently used unnecessary force on tissue or caused damage by inappropriate use of instruments		Careful handling of tissue but occasionally caused inadvertent damage		Consistently handled tissue appropriately with minimal damage to tissue

Time and motion

1	2	3	4	5
Many unnecessary moves		Efficient time/motion but some unnecessary moves		Clear economy of movement and maximum efficiency

Instrument handling

1	2	3	4	5
Repeatedly makes tentative or awkward moves with instruments through inappropriate use		Competent use of instruments but occasionally appeared stiff or awkward		Fluid movements with instruments and no stiffness or awkwardness

Knowledge of instruments

1	2	3	4	5
Frequently asked for wrong instrument or used inappropriate instrument		Knew names of most instruments and used appropriate instrument		Obviously familiar with instruments and their names

Flow of operation

1	2	3	4	5
Frequently stopped operating and seemed unsure of next move		Demonstrated some forward planning and reasonable progression of procedure		Obviously planned course of operation with effortless flow from one move to the next

Use of assistants

1	2	3	4	5
Consistently placed assistants poorly or failed to use assistants		Appropriate use of assistants most of the time		Strategically used assistants to the best advantage

Knowledge of specific procedure

1	2	3	4	5
Deficient knowledge. Required specific instructions at most steps		Knew all important steps of operation		Demonstrated familiarity with all steps of operation

OVERALL PERFORMANCE

1	2	3	4	5
Very poor		Competent		Clearly superior

QUALITY OF FINAL PRODUCT

1	2	3	4	5
Very poor		Competent		Clearly superior

In an attempt to further validate the OSATS, Faulkner and colleagues[9] performed a study wherein the scores in OSATS examinations were compared with surgeons' opinions about the residents' technical skills. This study confirmed that faculty are able to discriminate between residents with a high degree of precision. Further, there is close correlation between the faculty's opinions about residents and their OSATS scores. The correlation increases with advancing levels of training. Reznick and colleagues[10] reported on a large-scale administration of the OSATS, which was aimed at investigating reliability and validity. Inter-station reliabilities in the 0.80 range were achieved for this examination. This level of reliability is satisfactory for using examination scores to make high-level decisions.

Further experimentation in this examination focused on the utility of using the final product of the surgical procedure as a measure of how well that procedure was done.[11] It appears that assessing the product has a high degree of predictive power. It alone accounts for 50 percent of the variability between scores.

The examination has been used across four schools in Ontario, Canada, looking specifically at its utility for assessing senior level trainees. At this level, the OSATS has a high level of reliability and a good level of construct validity. It appears that the examination, as it exists, can be used at the certification level.

Since this examination requires a large amount of preparation and a cadre of knowledgeable individuals, a recent project was undertaken to assess the portability of the examination. A Toronto-based team, using a model of central administration and peripheral delivery, administered the examination to residents-in-training in Los Angeles and Chicago. This effort proved that the examination could be run at distant sites while maintaining its psychometric properties.

To be sure, this examination format is labour-intensive and expensive. It costs approximately $200.00 (CDN) per resident, per iteration. This figure does not include the substantial amount of faculty time (at each administration) nor the funds that have gone into its research and development.

The examination also requires a dedicated faculty who serve as examiners. However, as with most examination formats, when one moves from a pencil and paper-based format to a performance-based format, costs rise exponentially. One could argue however that the increased cost is paying for a more valid form of assessment.

SUMMARY

A great deal of effort is being spent on the acquisition of feasible, valid, and reliable instruments for the assessment of technical skill. Such instruments are necessary adjuncts in the training of technical skills and they help to ensure some level of quality control in the system of training. Standardisation of the evaluation environment is a key component of the evaluation of complex tasks. It allows increased reliability of measurement and permits meaningful comparisons between trainees both within and between levels of training. It is impossible to standardise the operating room environment enough to achieve a reliable measurement of technical skill, so technical skill assessment must be taken to a different venue. For the purpose of testing, bench simulations using fabricated models have been a reasonable substitute for the operating room environment. Bench models avoid the problems encountered with the use of cadavers and live animals, although the fidelity of anatomic reproduction requires ongoing research.

The use of checklists helps to objectify the measurement of complex tasks by breaking the task into simpler skills that are each rated separately and summed to achieve a score for the task. This component approach is also useful for providing detailed feedback to residents and to training programs. Global rating forms that are properly anchored with descriptors and used by trained evaluators in a standard testing situation have also been shown to be quite reliable measurement instruments. However, global rating forms measure more complex behaviours rather than simple tasks and are useful partners to the checklist forms in achieving meaningful evaluation of technical skill.

The Surgical Education Group at the University of Toronto has combined bench model simulation with checklists and global rating forms to achieve a feasible, reliable and valid method of technical skills assessment. The OSATS is also very useful for candidate and program feedback.

There remains much investigation to be done in the quest to improve technical skills testing. New technology, techniques and materials can be adopted to increase the fidelity of the testing environment. Virtual reality systems promise to improve realism while maintaining control of the testing situation for standardisation of measurement. Currently, however, the systems lack enough detail to be applicable. Haptic or force-feedback instruments are being developed to work with virtual reality systems as a means of interfacing the computerised environment with the candidate. The force feedback instruments give the candidate tactile information that increases the realism of the simulation. However, the widespread implementation of technical skills testing cannot wait for the perfection of these new techniques. The public and the profession demand that surgeons be properly trained and this can only be assured with good assessment of technical skills.

References

1.   Spencer CF. Teaching and measuring surgical techniques – the technical evaluation of competence. *Bull Am Coll Surg* 1978; 63:9-12.

2.   Barnes RW. Surgical handicraft: teaching and learning surgical skills. *Amer J Surg* 1987;153:422-27.

3.   Rutkow I *Surgery: An Illustrated History,* St. Louis, MO: Mosby Publishing; 1993.

4.   Kopta JA. An approach to the evaluation of operative skills. *Surg* 1971; 70:297-303.

5.   Stotter AT, Becket AJ, *et al.* Simulation in surgical training using freeze-dried material. *Br J Surg* 1986; 73:52-54.

6.   Bevan PG. The anastomosis workshop. *Ann R Coll Surg Eng* 1981; 63:405-10.

7.   Winckel CP, Reznick RK, Cohen R, *et al.* Reliability and construct validity of a structured technical skills assessment form. *Am J Surg* 1994; 167:423-27.

8.   Martin, JA, Regehr G, Reznick RK, *et al.* Objective structured assessment of technical skill (OSATS) for surgical residents. *Br J Surg* 1997; 84:273-78.

9.   Faulkner H, Regehr G, Martin J, *et al.* Validation of an objective structured assessment of technical skill for surgical residents. *Acad Med* 1996; 71:1363-65.

10.   Reznick RK, Regehr G, MacRae H, *et al.* Testing technical skill via an innovative 'Bench Station' examination. *Am J Surg* 1997; 173:226-30.

11.   Regehr G, MacRae H, Reznick RK. Comparing the psychometric properties of checklists and global rating scales for assessing performance on an OSCE-format examination. *Acad Med* 1998; 73:993-97.

Communication Skills for Surgeons: the Need for Assessment

Dr Patricia Wilkie

Chairman of the Patients Liaison Group, Royal College of General Practitioners
and Royal College of Radiologists.

Abstract

In this short paper, the importance of good communication skills for surgeons has been emphasised. These skills can be taught. Good communication by surgeons can have a direct effect on improved post-operative care and rehabilitation as well as on the quality of the relationship between surgeon and patient which is to the benefit of all. The assessment of communication skills is difficult. The different methods of assessment that can be used in teaching, in examination and in revalidation are discussed. The challenge for the profession is how and when to involve lay people in the assessment process.

At first glance it may not seem obvious why there should be a presentation on the assessment of communication skills in surgeons at a major conference on surgical competence.

Patients, their relatives and carers assume that they will receive information about the treatments available and the treatment options.[1] Many patients now expect to receive not only information given to them verbally by the doctor they are consulting but also for this information to be supported by a variety of written and other material.

More than 30 years ago, Cartwright's research[2] showed that 60% of patients interviewed mentioned some failure in communication. In 1999, problems in communication remain the most common cause of dissatisfaction and complaints made to health authorities, Trusts, voluntary organisations and community health councils. Stewart[3] systematically reviewed studies of patient-doctor communication and concluded that effective communication was often positively associated with improved patient outcomes: in physical, emotional and functional terms.

GIVING INFORMATION

It is, therefore, likely that the quality of information received by the patient may well affect the relationship between patients and doctor. The General Medical Council (GMC) in its document *Good Medical Practice*[4] describes successful relationships between doctors and patients as depending on trust. To establish and maintain that trust, doctors must:
■ give patients the information they ask for or need about their condition, its treatment and prognosis;
■ give information to patients in a way that they can understand it;
■ be satisfied that wherever possible the patient has understood what is proposed and consents to it before treatment is provided or investigations carried out; and
■ respect the right of patients to be fully involved in decisions about their care.

The giving of information appropriate to the needs of individual patients is not always easy. Patients are all different. They do, however, have one thing in common. Most are, if not frightened, at least apprehensive when meeting a surgeon. And this fear may affect their ability to understand what is being said to them making the work of the surgeon even more difficult. Many of the studies that have examined communications between doctors and patients have shown that:
■ patients often do not know the meaning of words used by clinicians;

■ patients have their own ideas about illness and these often differ from the medical model; and

■ patients often fail to understand what they are told by medial staff.[5]

There are many possible explanations for these problems in communication. The patient's apprehension has already been mentioned. Doctors use technical language and even at times a shorthand form of technical language and may have great difficulty in considering how these concepts can be explained to a patient. Medical terms such as 'venous cannulation' and 'serial bloods' are unlikely to be familiar to the majority of patients, many of whom have a very hazy idea of their own anatomy.[6] The specialist language and technical terms so familiar to professionals in their everyday work may be incomprehensible to even intelligent lay people. Surgeons are busy people and little, if any, time appears to be set aside for communication. Furthermore, what the patient has been told does not appear to be routinely recorded in the notes as would be a laboratory result, thus increasing the possibility of poor communication and mixed messages between patient and staff.

The tone and manner in which the information is delivered are also important and may affect the patient's understanding. Few patients address the doctor in the manner in which they are spoken to. Care needs to be taken so that the patient is not 'talked down' to. When we become patients, we are vulnerable and may not wish to admit that we do not understand.

COMMUNICATION SKILLS

The need for good communication skills is essential, as surgeons must obtain consent from patients for investigations and treatments. The GMC[7] states that patients have a right to information about their condition and the treatment options available to them. This should include:

■ the nature of the condition;

■ the complexity of the treatment;

■ the risks associated with the procedure;

■ the short- and long-term implications of the procedure;

■ the purpose of the investigation or procedure;

■ how the patient should prepare for the procedure; and

■ what the patient may experience after the procedure.

It is clear that it is now essential that surgeons acquire good communication skills. These skills include:

■ the ability to explain complex information to patient in a manner that they understand;

■ an understanding and awareness of lay concepts of disease;

■ the ability to listen to the patient;

■ an understanding and awareness of possible social, religious and cultural differences which could impede comprehension;

■ an understanding and awareness of non-verbal communication and body language;

■ an understanding and awareness of factors such as lack of privacy, noise etc, which can prevent good communication; and

■ knowledge of written and other information which could help the patient.

This is not a comprehensive list. It is simply intended to give a flavour of the dimensions of the components that need to be used in good communication. However skilled in other aspects of their work, the great majority of surgeons have something to learn from a course in communication skills. It is encouraging that the Competence Assessment Working Party set up by the Joint Committee on Higher Surgical Training which oversees surgical training in all surgical specialities in the United Kingdom and the Republic of Ireland under the chairmanship of Professor Galasko, has included communication skills as one of the skills that a trainee must have. These skills, therefore, need to be taught and then competency assessed.

METHODS OF ASSESSMENT

There are a variety of ways in which communication skills can be assessed including:
■ assessment of the student during a communication skills course;
■ observation of an actual consultation;
■ observation of a simulated consultation involving actors;
■ analysis of a video-recorded consultation; and
■ evaluation by patients.

Each of these methods have their advantages and disadvantages and more than one method can be used for any assessment. All participants in a communication skills course should be assessed and in the future it is hoped that all surgeons will participate in such courses. The advantages of assessment on a course is that participants can be assessed using different methods of assessment and over a period of time.

Direct observation of a surgeon communicating with a patient has the advantage of observing how the person conducts themselves. The disadvantages are that the presence of another person can be intrusive for the patient and may also change the dynamics of the consultation.

The use of a simulated consultation with appropriately trained and briefed actors taking the place of patients is adopted in some communication skills courses. The student can be faced with many different scenarios decided by the tutor. The scenario can be repeated in areas where a student is having difficulties and patients are not inconvenienced. This type of simulation can be a very good training method. The disadvantage is that the situation is artificial and the 'unpredictability' of a communication between a patient and a surgeon is not replicated.

Video-recorded consultations provide detailed information about the student's ability to communicate. This is both a good teaching and assessment method. The permission of the patients does need to be sought. The experience of the Royal College of General Practitioners is that this does not present a problem providing the video is only being used for educational purposes. Video recording does not involve a third person and the actual consultation is observed. The disadvantage is that expensive equipment is required, possibly in a fixed location.

An evaluation, in the form of a questionnaire, of what patients have understood can be a very useful way of assessing aspects of communication skills. It may be easier to evaluate in situations where a precise set of information and facts has been given. The advantage of such a method is that direct feedback from the patient can be gained; the difficulty is to get the timing right. The patient needs to have time to assimilate the information but not to have forgotten it. Questionnaires need to be well focused and preferably validated. Disadvantages include the difficulties of finding an appropriate questionnaire and response rate.

ASSESSORS

Whichever methods of assessment are used, the criteria for assessment need to be developed and the assessors trained. The teaching of communication skills to doctors is frequently undertaken by psychologists and other social scientists, as well as by doctors with a particular interest in this subject. The examining or testing of communication skills should be carried out by examiners experienced in this subject.

The assessment of communication skills should also be a component in the process of revalidation of surgeons. This process could include lay assessors.

CONCLUSION

In this short paper, the importance of good communication skills for surgeons has been emphasised. These skills can be taught. Good communication by surgeons can have a direct effect on improved post- operative care and rehabilitation, as well as on the quality of the relationship between surgeon and doctor which is to the benefit of all. The assessment of communication skills is difficult. Different methods of assessment can be used in teaching, in examination and in revalidation. Finally, the challenge for the profession is how and when to involve lay people in the assessment process.

References

1.   Wilkie P. The expectations of the modern patient. *Proc R Coll Physicians Edinb* 1996; 26:575-580.

2.   Stewart M. Effective physician-patient communication and health outcomes: a review. *Canadian Medical Assoc Journal* 1995; 152:1423-33.

3.   Cartwright A. *Human Relations and Hospital Care.* Oxford: Routledge & Kegan Paul; 1964.

4.   General Medical Council. *Good Medical Practice.* London: GMC Publications; 1998.

5.   Tuckett D, Boulton M, Olson C, Williams A. *Meeting Between Experts: An Approach to Sharing Ideas in Medical Consultations.* London: Tavistock; 1985.

6.   Wilkie P. The patient perspective. In: Sims J, ed. *Primary Health Care Sciences.* London: Whurr Publishers; 1999.

7.   General Medical Council. *Seeking Patients' Consent: The Ethical Considerations.* London: GMC Publications; 1998.

Proficiency Training
for Space Flight

Frank E Hughes

NASA/Space Flight Training Division (retired)

Abstract

Training for space flight on the space shuttle is extremely complex. Each astronaut is faced with enormous amounts of material that must be mastered. Specialised simulators are utilised to assist the crew in learning that material. Knowledge must also be maintained so that the student astronaut remains in a state of flight readiness. Since shuttle flight duration is short, proficiency is not an issue during such flights. However, the gaps between flights can be quite lengthy, and so proficiency training is utilised to insure that the crews maintain the highest state of readiness.

With the arrival of the International Space Station, proficiency becomes an issue due to the possibility of flights of extremely long duration. Maintaining proficiency thus becomes increasingly challenging. Various remedies such as refresher training provide an 'on demand' opportunity for each person to request additional training pre-launch. In addition, onboard training will be utilised to ensure that the crew remains viable during their flight. The challenge of proficiency training is for the training managers to determine how much and how often it should be applied in order to ensure safe flight operations.

When a crew of astronauts is selected to fly the space shuttle, it is the culmination of a long series of training events that are remarkably thorough. Astronauts are selected from two special groups of people. The pilot astronauts are jet pilots in the military services of the United States (Air Force, Navy, and Marines) who have excelled in their careers within the operational squadrons. Test pilot schools select the pilots from within their service for further training. Applicants to NASA are forwarded by each service based on their performance following graduation from either Patuxet River NAS Test Pilot School or Edwards AFB Test Pilot School. Needless to say, they are excellent pilots. NASA interviews 20 or 30 of these pilots and selects 10 or 12 each year to begin training for shuttle flights.

CANDIDATES

The second set of candidates is all graduate scientists or engineers, doctors, dentists, or veterinarians. These individuals must have at least three years of experience post-graduation. Interestingly enough, they do not have to have an advanced degree. (However, since about 8,000 persons continuously have applications on file, every time NASA issues a call for applicants, degrees rapidly become discriminators for selection.) These candidates must have excelled in their field and have impressed their superiors and peers. Then they must pass the same selection process as the pilots. This is a battery of tests, which includes a series of face-to-face interviews with senior NASA personnel (including current astronauts) before selection is made.

SELECTION

Selection into NASA's astronaut program means starting a one-year candidacy period in which nearly 1,000 hours of instruction is provided. This instruction covers all of the important systems operation of the shuttle and space station, flight instruction in a high-performance jet aircraft (for the non-pilots), and various utilitarian classes such as 'how to handle the press'. The performance of the student in these classes is critical since it is from the graduates of these courses that future flight crews will be selected.

Following this year of candidacy, the person graduates as an astronaut ready for flight assignment. Once assignment occurs, more training is provided which is 'mission specific' in nature; that is, it builds on the previously given generic training by focusing on specific operations for the upcoming flight. This training can take up to 18 months but averages about nine months. An entire crew of five to seven persons goes through this training, as a group for the most part and individually as necessary. The flight commander and training manager are responsible for ensuring that all the training for the flight is accomplished. The actual training lessons are extracted from the official Shuttle Training Catalogue. It is during this period of training that a need for proficiency training is first encountered.

SIMULATORS

Most of the training time, however, is spent in the various simulators that ingrain classroom knowledge more deeply in the student. They allow a student to practice extremely detailed processes and then repeat them again and again to ensure skill development and retention. The use of simulators was pioneered by NASA years ago to allow pilots to perform various space activities that were too complicated, too costly and too dangerous to do otherwise. Simulator building is a fine art now and NASA is moving rapidly away from large and costly simulators to small flexible devices that incorporate virtual environments where possible.

All of the training lessons for shuttle or station are detailed within a catalogue not unlike the one utilised for most colleges. Every course and lesson is detailed in this document. The planned training is listed along with the duration of the class, any prerequisites and a short lesson synopsis. The individual lessons are graphed into a sequence that is shown as Figure 1. These represent what the astronauts call 'training flows'. The details of each lesson in the flow is shown as a specific page in the catalogue where all of the detailed information is provided. Within this catalogue and its flows, it also shows whether proficiency training is needed for a given skill taught in that lesson.

At this point, definitions are needed for three terms that are closely related and which form the basis for this paper. The terms are proficiency training, refresher training and just-in-time training. These terms are similar in concept and are chiefly distinguished by frequency of occurrence, by qualification or currency maintenance issues and by whether you are introducing new material versus previously taught material.

The definitions of the terms are:

Proficiency Training – training scheduled on a recurring basis throughout the training process to ensure the maintenance and retention of previously acquired knowledge, skills, or attitudes with respect to specific tasks.

Refresher Training – training conducted on an as-needed basis at the request of an individual crew member to cover topics of interest to the student.

Just-in-Time Training – new skills training that is conducted following initial qualification training, and immediately prior to specific task execution.

Figure 1. Example of a 'training flow'

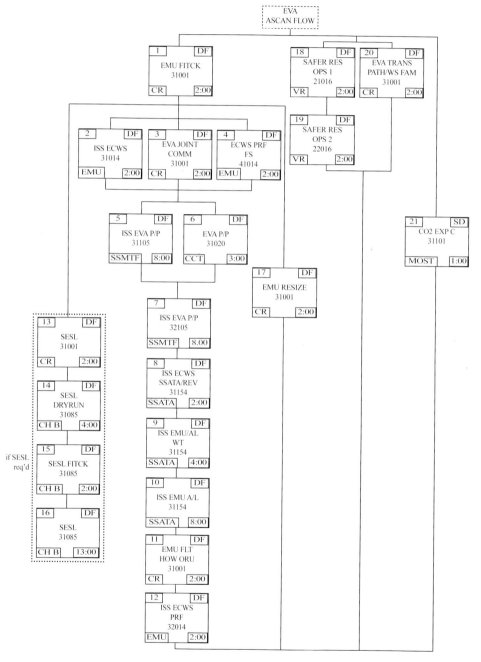

EMU Systems Flow

Proficiency training

Proficiency training applies to International Space Station systems, payload and vehicle training. It is used to maintain crew performance levels according to program requirements. Either the payload development or flight operations team may levy requirements for proficiency training. It is scheduled on a recurring basis throughout the training process to ensure the maintenance and retention of previously acquired knowledge, skills or attitudes with respect to specific tasks. This type of training is not used to introduce new knowledge, skills or attitudes. Ground-based proficiency training requirements are defined in the respective crew-training flows and are scheduled by the crew-training manager. This type of training has a high priority on simulator scheduling. The reason is that NASA feels that it saves valuable simulator time later to use some of the initial training time for proficiency. Proficiency training is also performed on-orbit using newly developed, small, PC-based simulators. Ground-based proficiency training is co-ordinated through the training manager, while proficiency training needed after launch is co-ordinated through personnel in Mission Control.

Proficiency training is usually required when there are long time spans between training and task execution. The maximum time span between training sessions or between training and operations is defined as the currency requirement. The training templates and schedules will adhere to these currency requirements in order to ensure that levels of crew proficiency are maintained. Orbit proficiency training time requirements may be less stringent than those used pre-flight, but cannot be more. The zero gravity (zero-g) environment may affect on-orbit proficiency training. If that turns out to be true, that will, in turn, influence the currency requirements. As operational experience with prolonged periods of zero-g increases, and the nature of space station operations becomes better understood, proficiency requirements for skills such as robotics and space-suited operations may be adjusted.

Proficiency requirements for payloads are identified during the training planning process. The requirements are then forwarded to the training manager for a particular increment, who will then include the requirements in the payload input to the training plan for that flight. Proficiency training that is required to be executed on-orbit will be taken out of the time allotted for that payload on-orbit. For this reason, payload investigators must submit on-orbit proficiency training requirements to their respective payload planners so that the planners understand the requirements thoroughly.

The need for proficiency training for generic knowledge, skills and attitudes is established through the crew training flow development process. Any advanced training proficiency requirements are documented in the generic training plan followed by all new astronauts.

For a specific space station increment, crew proficiency training is defined in the crew-training flow and reflected in the training plan for those systems and payload proficiency requirements that are specific to that flight. Monthly practice for space-suited operations is an example of regularly scheduled proficiency training.

Refresher training

Refresher training is training conducted on an as-needed basis at the request of an individual crew member and after consultation with appropriate training personnel. In this case, the student astronaut may request additional simulator time or simply tutorials. Refresher training, although not required at specified intervals, is generally taken if it has been a significant length of time since the original training. This training is typically used to review and stimulate each crew member's knowledge and understanding of space station systems, payloads and vehicles as well as their associated skills. The refresher lessons may be repeats of previous lessons or a combination of several lessons. Because the need for refresher training is dependent upon individual crew members, the training organisations responsible for the training execution and the requesting crew member will consult to determine appropriate content of the training and which simulator is to be used. As with proficiency training, this type of training is not used to provide new material.

Just-in-time training

Just-in-time training is defined as any training session that is conducted following initial qualification training, and immediately prior to specific task execution. Since most crews prefer to train and practice as many of the required tasks as possible prior to launch, just-in-time training will generally be limited to unanticipated tasks. However, in the future there will surely be an increase in the amount of just-in-time training used on a given flight. New training material is a distinguishing characteristic of just-in-time training since it involves the presentation of previously untrained material. Just-in-time training is possible both as ground- and on-orbit-based training. Ground-based just-in-time training may be used when it is necessary to change the assigned crew person for a specific increment. It could also be utilised when user interface changes are made to computer displays, and as necessary equipment upgrades are made. Circumstances that may warrant on-orbit just-in-time training are unanticipated hardware maintenance tasks and crew healthcare emergencies. Just-in-time training is a powerful tool but it must be utilised appropriately to avoid providing less than adequate crew training for specific tasks.

Thus, a shuttle flight training plan consists of a series of planned lessons out of the catalogue with adequate time for each crew member to request and accomplish any refresher training they desire. Proficiency training in the simulators is used to maintain each person's skills up to the day those skills are required. As much training as possible is waived in lieu of just-in-time training to minimise the total training which the crew must endure either singly or as a group. The utilisation of each of these types of training allows the length of the training to be as short as possible.

In any business enterprise or profession, the applicability of any or all of these proficiency or refresher training methods depends heavily on what kind of activity is under discussion. Basically, proficiency and refresher would be widely applicable in many disciplines but just-in-time training might have a narrower application scope. It is clear that you would want your airline pilots to have as much refresher training as they might want. It would also be clear that there should be certain minimum proficiency maintenance activities required of all pilots. (And there are such rules within all of the airlines as well as very accurate simulators to implement them.) But it would be disturbing, to say the least, if the pilot on your plane was to utilise just-in-time training for anything to do with taking off or landing that aeroplane!

APPLICATION

It is also clear that the applicability of these concepts is highly interrelated with the utilisation of simulators and simulation techniques. As the use of small, low-cost simulators increases (with virtual environments integrated into them), the possibility of proficiency examinations and tests becomes much more likely. Experimental surgical activities, using virtual environments, at the NASA/Johnson Space Centre and other locations have indicated that this is a potentially viable field.

CONCLUSION

The usefulness of virtual surgery in the university situation is obvious and needs to be developed further immediately. However, once available, it would be imperative to increase the utilisation of this technique for proficiency training in many areas. The hospital situation would be a perfect place to utilise this technique. The ability to have a surgeon perform a procedure on demand from some oversight panel would be extremely beneficial assuming that the technical problems can be remedied. Such a test would allow the oversight group to observe the doctor in question and to evaluate the skills that the governing body had chosen to be necessary for candidates for certification.

Certain microsurgical procedures such as those utilising fibre-optical techniques lend themselves to virtual surgical training. In these areas, the surgeon is already encumbered with the technical equipment necessary to perform the operation itself. Adding a virtual source for the visible scene within which the doctor is operating would be a small inconvenience as long as the visibility and realism reached adequate levels. Other types of virtual surgery (ie occurring in a regular operating theatre) might require more equipment or larger databases and the realism would be more difficult to achieve.

More research must occur at this time to determine just how much skill transfer a surgeon can expect from a virtual operating room situation. The future of any serious proficiency training for medical personnel must include the ability to utilise simulated situations and equipment that includes haptic or touch feedback to the student. The sense of touch is one of the most critical in this environment and it is the least developed in today's virtual equipment. The ability to handle real trauma situations and learn procedures in a virtual world would be optimal for any new medical students. The students would be able to perform the required surgical tasks in a safe and non-threatening environment. The tutorial capabilities this technique would provide would be extremely useful in increasing the efficiency of the training process. This idea of virtual surgery would bring to the medical profession the same proficiency tools that aid today's pilots and astronauts. The benefits from the application of this new technology could prove to be tremendous.

Reading list

1.   Virtual Environments: http://www.vetl.uh.edu/
        http://www.vetl.uh.edu/ScienceSpace/Pics/gallery.html

2.   Virtual Medical Operations: http://www.vetl.uh.edu/surgery/surpage.html

3.   Simulators: http://www.hq.nasa.gov/office/pao/History/computers/Ch9-2.html
        http://ails.arc.nasa.gov/Images/InfoSys/AC96-0210-9.html

Challenges in Developing and Maintaining Skills and Proficiency

Carolyn L Huntoon PhD

Assistant Secretary for Environmental Management at the Department of Energy, USA

Arnauld E Nicogossian MD

Abstract

NASA utilises a number of vehicles to deliver training and maintain the proficiency of astronauts. The first step NASA has developed is the selection process for new astronauts, ensuring that they initially have a certain level of knowledge and competency. Through the use of simulators and mock-ups, NASA further increases and refines this knowledge base. The methodologies for astronaut training are based in the military approach, reflecting NASA's early use of military personnel as astronauts. It is nearly impossible to reproduce the microgravity environment encountered in space flight on Earth. Therefore, NASA's training facilities simulate aspects of the space environment. Astronauts are trained to be familiar with all the systems on the spacecraft and to have specialised knowledge about biomedical science, engineering, astronomy, or physical science. NASA supplements computer-based training with virtual reality enhanced techniques, providing immersive, interactive training displays.

This technique also allows individuals from distant locations to train or work together in the same virtual environment, real-time. The final supplement to training discussed in this paper is the use of telemedicine to connect space travelling physicians and technicians to ground-based experts and ground support teams. Future applications of NASA-developed technology include three-dimensional visualisations in virtual clinics and virtual surgery to enhance skills before actually donning scrubs.

INTRODUCTION

Similar to the way medical schools select and train students, NASA has evolved a system for selecting and training astronauts that relies on a number of management approaches. Initially, NASA selects individuals who meet certain pre-set criteria in terms of education and experience. Secondly, they undergo a twelve-month intensive study of science, engineering and space flight systems. It is only then that NASA designates them astronauts. The individual is assigned to a particular mission, usually based on aligning mission objectives with education, experience of the potential space traveller and crew compatibility, then intensive training for science missions begins. This training lasts from nine to 18 months. The various types of training – proficiency, refresher or just-in-time – that NASA offers to the astronaut corps are discussed in the previous chapter by Frank Hughes. This paper addresses the challenges of developing and maintaining skills and proficiencies.[1, 2]

There is a similarity between the challenges NASA overcomes in training astronauts and the difficulty in training surgeons. Astronauts train under conditions that are familiar and gravity – based, however they perform tasks in a radically different environment, microgravity, surrounded by a near vacuum. Similarly, surgeons do not train under the same conditions that they encounter in the operating room. To train space crews, NASA has developed a suite of simulators and facilities which mimic various aspects of the space environment. However, the first time the actual task is performed in space is the first time that the astronaut has all the elements with which to contend.

SELECTION OF SPACE CREWS

Medical schools select students who demonstrate intelligence and stamina and who are trainable. Approximately every two years, NASA conducts an astronaut selection. There are two categories of individuals that are examined, pilots and mission specialists. To be considered for pilot positions, applicants must have extensive experience in high performance jet aircraft and mission specialist applicants must have significant backgrounds in engineering, physical or life sciences. Selection occurs after a lengthy process of personal interviews, background investigations and medical evaluations. The first astronauts were from the military and all had jet aircraft flight experience and engineering training. This early experience has carried forward into the training regimens today, leaving a military influence on the conduct of training. It was not until 1964 that educational background was a consideration in selection rather than just military experience.[3]

Today's applicants usually have an advanced degree in one or more fields and at least three years' relevant experience in engineering, biological science, physical science or mathematics. After extensive evaluation of the entire applicant pool, the highly qualified undergo a week-long evaluation process of personal interviews and medical evaluations. A panel of experts recommends acceptance based on the education, training, experience, unique qualifications and skills. The several hundred applicants that fulfil the requirements are evaluated on their ability to be team players with just the right amount of individuality and self-reliance to be effective crew members. Once selected, the applicant is designated as an astronaut candidate and assigned to the astronaut office for a one-year training and evaluation period.

During this year of training, astronaut candidates receive information on systems they will encounter as career astronauts such as Shuttle systems, basic science, technology, mathematics, geology, meteorology, guidance and navigation, oceanography, orbital dynamics, astronomy, physics and materials processing. They also receive training in parachute jumping, land and sea survival, and scuba diving. Candidates study the problems associated with space suits, high (hyperbaric) and low (hypobaric) atmospheric pressures, and emergencies. They are exposed to the microgravity of space flight in a modified KC-135 jet aircraft that produces periods of weightlessness for 20 seconds as it dives from an altitude of 35,000 to 24,000 feet. Pilot astronauts also maintain flying proficiency by flying 15 hours per month in NASA's fleet of two-seat T-38 jets. Upon completion of this year, they may be designated astronauts. There have been 276 astronauts who have been selected and trained by this regimen and have flown in space for the US program.

ASTRONAUT FORMAL TRAINING

To overcome the inability to actually reproduce the microgravity environment of space, NASA uses simulators in astronaut training. Initially, the single systems trainer, a mock-up of the space shuttle systems, is used. Subsequently, the astronauts begin training in the complex Shuttle Mission Simulators which simulate all areas of Shuttle vehicle operations and in all flight phases: pre-launch, ascent, orbital, entry and landing. Missions can be simulated literally from launch to landing using a digital image generation system to provide visual cues for out-the-window scenes of the entire mission, such as the Earth, stars, payloads, or the landing runway. These simulated missions can take place on a fixed-base or motion-based platform. The fixed-base crew station is used for mission and payload training, launch, descent and landing training. The motion base crew station is used to train pilots and commanders in launch, descent and landing, using a 6-degrees-of-freedom motion system. Total hours in the Shuttle Mission Simulator for the astronauts, after flight assignment, is about 300 hours.

Several part-task trainers are used to prepare astronauts for particular aspects of the mission. The primary facility used to train individuals to perform extravehicular activities, called EVAs, is the Sonny Carter Training Facility. This is a 62 million-gallon pool, measuring 102 by 202 by 40 feet, that provides neutral buoyancy similar to the weightless environment that is experienced by spacecraft and crew during space flight. The astronaut, wearing a modified space suit, trains to perform EVA operations in this simulated zero-g environment that mimics the dynamics of body motion under weightless conditions. This training is conducted on full size mock-ups, which are also submerged. In addition to EVA tasks, astronauts perform intravehicular activities, called IVAs.

To train for IVAs, space crews utilise many facilities depending on the task such as maintenance of the spacecraft both planned and unforeseen, payload set-up and operation, use of various special tools, housekeeping, exercise and health maintenance. Full-scale mock-ups and trainers are used for onboard-systems orientation and habitability training in such things as meal preparation, equipment stowage, trash management, camera use and experiment familiarisation.

This full-scale mock-up is also used to train for a possible emergency exit during a landing. The crew compartment trainer is a mock-up of the forward section of the orbiter, without a payload bay, that can be tilted vertically, simulating the configuration of the shuttle just before launch. The manipulator development facility is a full-scale mock-up of the payload bay with a full-scale hydraulically operated mechanical arm, used to move payloads in and out of the payload bay. This facility is used to train astronauts to move objects into, out of, and around the payload bay, without performing an EVA or in some cases to assist with an EVA.

Pilots receive more intensive instruction in orbiter approach and landing in Shuttle Training Aircraft (STA), which are four Gulfstream II business jets modified to perform like the orbiter during landing. Because the Orbiter approaches landings at such a steep angle (17-20 degrees) and high speed (over 300 miles per hour), the STA approaches with its engines in reverse thrust and main landing gear down to increase drag and duplicate the unique glide characteristics of the orbiter. Assigned pilots receive about 100 hours of STA training prior to a flight, which is equivalent to 600 Shuttle approaches. The first real shuttle landing by each commander is after returning from spaceflight lasting from four to 16 days. As the time from STA training to the actual landing increases, the pilot astronaut uses an onboard computer to maintain proficiency in performing landing tasks.

In between training sessions, the crew members continue to keep themselves up-to-date on the status of the spacecraft and payloads for their assigned mission. In addition, the astronauts study flight rules and flight data file procedures, and participate in mission-related technical meetings. They also participate in test and check-out activities at the NASA Kennedy Space Centre in Florida, the launch site for the Space Shuttle.

Astronauts often comment that only the noise and vibration of launch and the experience of weightlessness are missing from the practice sessions; everything else in training accurately duplicates the space experience. After the Orbiter has returned, the crew will spend several days debriefing and recounting their experiences for the benefit of future crews to assist in future training and to add to the space flight knowledge base.

VIRTUAL REALITY TRAINING FACILITIES

The Virtual Environment Technology Laboratory (VETL), developed in conjunction with the University of Houston, is used for teaching and training. Virtual reality, an immersive, spatially expansive training environment, complements NASA's more traditional computer-based teaching systems with intelligent, virtual environments that are interactive. The VETL technology is available to the private sector and industries throughout the Houston region, concentrating on the use of virtual environment technology in oil, gas and medicine.

The VETL, using high performance graphics hardware and software, displays the visual components of virtual environments on monitors, stereoscopic head-mounted displays, and projection displays. The three-dimensional visualisation of applications such as seismic interpretations, simulations of production platforms, and geophysical models of hydrocarbon reservoirs, allows multiple users to simultaneously analyse complex data. Application of this technology eliminates the need to bring together personnel from distant locations for training or data analysis at a central location. Individuals in multiple locations spanning the globe are able to train or work together in the same virtual environment with near real-time interaction. For example, astronauts located in both Houston, Texas and Darmstadt, Germany trained to repair a satellite recently. Chemists at the University of Houston and the University of California at San Diego directly collaborate by immersively exploring and manipulating large molecular structures together without leaving their laboratories.[4]

The space mission to repair the Hubble Space Telescope (HST) was one of the most procedurally complex space missions to be executed in years. Virtual reality played a significant role in training the many people involved with making the mission a success. In order to transfer knowledge of the HST hardware and EVA procedures, the training addressed both cognitive and psychomotor skills. Before entering the virtual HST environment, the learner already had basic knowledge of the hardware components and task procedures from previous experiences and document study. The virtual environment therefore provided them with a three-dimensional view of what they had previously seen only in two-dimensional drawings or photographs. An important consideration in performing various steps has to do with an astronaut's orientation to the hardware item. In the virtual training environment, the astronaut manoeuvres with six degrees of freedom and experiences this orientation first-hand, gaining a better understanding of the psychomotor and visualisation skills required.[5]

The applications of virtual reality to enhancing surgical skills are relatively unexplored. A study conducted by the Institute for Defense Analyses evaluated the effectiveness of virtual reality as a surgical skills simulation tool for training.[6] The authors of the report determined that virtual reality simulation could duplicate the operative field, enhance training and reduce the need for expensive animal training models. Their hypothesis was that virtual reality in combination with fuzzy logic would be useful in educating surgeons and determining their competence to perform procedures on patients. The specific procedure they studied was laparoscopic surgery. The study was designed in two phases. Phase one was to determine the necessary skills of experienced surgeons required for technical competence. This determination was made by analysing surgical tasks and soliciting the input of subject matter experts. During the second phase of the project, researchers determined the capabilities of a virtual reality surgical skills simulator, by performing a series of simulator-based trials with both experienced and beginning surgeons, recording their psychomotor performance with skill-level tests, and measuring the simulator's ability to provide skill level training.[7]

Other research has indicated that instructional technology is an effective method for learning a variety of tasks and skills that produces savings in time, people, costs, and materials. Some researchers have suggested that virtual reality might provide an opportunity to introduce new training techniques and technologies to the field of medical education. Medical schools and hospitals would have new measurement tools to record and evaluate human psychomotor performance in specific surgical tasks.

SUPPLEMENTING NASA'S TRAINING REGIMEN

In addition to specific training on physiological monitoring of healthy crew members and medical care of ill or injured crew, NASA supplements the training of the ground support team of physicians and the physician astronauts with expert assistance from ground-based specialists. This expertise is accessed using NASA's telemedicine capabilities. NASA is credited with developing the first telemedicine project; in 1958, a South American squirrel monkey, Old Reliable, was launched 300 miles into space and the technical and scientific information on the physiological and behaviour status of the animal was gained through telemetry.[8] The medical monitors for the flight of Alan Shepard, Jr, the first American in space, included evaluating his medical status and correlating spacecraft data and physiological data with the mission profile.[9] By 1962 when John Glenn made three orbits of the Earth, NASA could rely on its own growing medical in-house capability and became less dependent upon the military services for medical support.[10]

NASA has continued to evolve telemedicine capabilities and applied the technologies and expertise on Earth for terrestrial healthcare, disaster management and extension of medical expertise to remote populations. Programs in which NASA has participated include:

■ Telemedicine Spacebridge to Armenia provided medical assistance in response to the December 7, 1988 earthquake in the Republic of Armenia, and the June 4, 1989 train/gas explosion accident in Ufa, Russia.

■ Space Bridge Moscow connected three medical centres in the US (LDS Hospital/University of Utah Health Sciences Centre, Salt Lake City, Utah; Fairfax Hospital, Falls Church, VA; and Yale University School of Medicine, New Haven, CT) to two medical centres in Moscow, Russia (Clinical Hospital of the Medical Department of the Ministry of Interior and the Moscow State University School of Medicine).

To monitor the physiological and medical impact of space flight on astronauts, NASA integrates telecommunications and medical technologies. During the past four decades NASA telemedicine technologies have found many applications in the delivery of healthcare on Earth. NASA is a recognised leader in telemedicine, working closely with other Federal agencies, industry and academia as well as its international partners.

Two-way voice communications and one-way video and data down-link comprise the main communications capabilities for conducting telemedicine. However, telemedicine has been applied to monitor environmental parameters, ensuring safe and comfortable ambient conditions and timely detection of any factors capable of interfering with health or performance of the crew. In-flight monitoring of medical data will play an even greater role in all phases of assembly and operation of the Space Station.

FUTURE DIRECTIONS

The International Space Station and our desire to explore the universe are driving NASA to advanced medical informatics. Ames Research Centre hosts the centre for Bioinformatics, which develops the advanced tools for NASA's medical care. An example of a future direction includes a virtual collaborative clinic which brings together physicians and technical staff located at remote sites that are able to interact with three-dimensional visualisations of patient-specific data. Recently the centre tested the system by performing a stereo reconstruction of a heart. Another development is the CyberScapel, which was used to demonstrate 3-D virtual jaw surgery. The surgical application is for irregular-shaped or round bones, organs, membrane-like structures (like the skull), and complex structures such as a mandible. This tool allows the surgeon to interact with the reconstruction to cut and manipulate desired regions of the skull.

The Virtual Environment for Reconstructive Surgery, is a collaboration between the Biocomputation Centre at NASA Ames Research Centre and the Department of Reconstructive Surgery at Stanford University. The intent is to produce an interactive, collaborative virtual environment for planning of craniofacial surgeries. A pilot project involves producing computer-based reconstructions of the facial structure of real patients then creating a virtual environment in which the surgeon may simulate and plan the operation.

CONCLUSION

Although NASA utilises many types of training to prepare astronauts to live and work in space, simulators play a vital role in the process. NASA is often cited for the state-of-the-art of its simulators. The use of virtual reality has provided another method of simulating the microgravity of space flight without actually launching a crew member. Telemedicine is employed to enhance the skills of the crew medical officer and other crew members through the use of ground-based experts as consultants.

Each of these methodologies builds on the manner in which crew persons are initially selected and have evolved from NASA's original links to the military. From this military background, training has been based on repetition. NASA has become proficient in determining a crew person's proficiency and in maintaining various skill sets between the time of training and practice sessions to the actual performance of a task. If this length of time is too great, NASA employs on-board computers to maintain skill level. This analogue can be applied to determining the readiness level of a physician to perform a given procedure initially and later to determine proficiency and retraining needs. The use of virtual reality as a training and refreshing tool has great potential both for NASA and to allow surgeons to plan and practice procedures.

References

1.   Project Mercury: Man-in-Space Program of the NASA. *Report # 1014, 86th Congress 1st Session.* Dec, 1959.

2.   Lovelace II WR, Schwichtenberg AH, Luft UC, and Secrest RR, Selection Find Maintenance Program for Astronauts for the National Aeronautics and Space Administration. *Aerospace Med;* 1962; 33(6):667-6334.

3.   Johnston R, Hayes EL, and Dietlein LF. *Crew Systems Development In Support of Manned Space Flight.* An undated manuscript circa summer 1963.

4.   Loftin RB. *Hands Across the Atlantic* (http://www.vetl.uh.edu/sharedvir/handatl.html)

5.   Loftin RB and Kenney PJ. Virtual Environments in Training: NASA's Hubble Space Telescope Mission. Presented at: 16th Interservice/Industry Training Systems & Education Conference; Nov 1994 Orlando, Florida.

6.   Johnston R *The Effectiveness of Instructional Technology: A Review of the Research.* Institute for Defense Analyses.

7.   Ota D, Loftin B, Saito T, Lea R, James Keller. *Virtual Reality in Surgical Education.* (http://www.vetl.uh.edu/surgery/vrse.html#contents)

8.   Van der Wal FL and Young WD. Project MIA (Mouse-in-Able), Experiments on physiological response to space flight. *ARS J.* 1959; 29(10):716-720.

9.   NASA Space Task Group Briefing. *Medical Monitoring for Project Mercury.* Dec 11, 1959.

10.   Aeronautical and Astronautical Events of 1961. *Report of the National Aeronautics and Space Administration to the Committee on Science and Astronautics.* US House of Representatives, 87th Cong 2nd sess. June 7 1962, p 68.

The Clinical Link

AW Goode MD FRCS

Professor of Endocrine and Metabolic Surgery
St Bartholomews and The Royal London Hospital School of Medicine and
Dentistry, London

Abstract

The manned spaceflight program has taken a central place in the public's perception of scientific competence and human endeavour. The accomplishment is built upon an understanding of the basic and intractable laws of physics and is an interaction of three elements, the crew, the spacecraft systems and the environment, with success dependent upon these elements being mutually supportive and properly integrated. NASA studies of the attributes of crew members and factors which produce a documented decrement in performance are comprehensive. With the evolution and complexity of manned spacecraft systems, the selection, training and support system have evolved to enhance and maintain standards and compatibility.

Ground base simulation is a key component of training and many aspects of it may be similar to the use of a simulator for the technical aspects of surgical procedures. There is, however, little evidence of its value in other aspects of surgical care. Certainly simulation may improve the performance of a trainee, but there are suggestions it is of limited value for the established practitioner. The identification of the underperforming practitioner is probably not possible with retrospective data analysis which is inherently unreliable. Just as a NASA mission simulation is an exercise in prospective evaluation, so too a mechanism will be suggested for a prospective assessment of surgical practice and a remedial mechanism for identified underperformance.

INTRODUCTION

Throughout time, man and circumstance have worked hand-in-hand to give substance to dreams. Christopher Columbus ventured to the edge of the sea to give us a New World, while William Harvey suffered ridicule and scientific ostracism for teaching the circulation for blood. Similarly, Van Leeuwenhoek's crude microscope upset fixed traditions of microbiology and Alexander Fleming's astute observations introduced a therapeutic revolution. All were events of profound significance driven in the main by the human traits of curiosity and enquiry combined with, in each case, historic circumstance and some specific aspect of the individual's character: physical bravery, mental resilience, state-of-the-art scientific exploitation and brilliant application of serendipity, respectively. To this tradition of adventure and discovery, following in the footsteps of Christopher Columbus, has been added government involvement, which has been the genesis of the manned spacecraft program, providing broad strategic aims while utilising the freedom of individual expertise.

Manned space flight may be viewed as an interaction of three particular elements:
- the crew member – identified by selection and training;
- the space craft systems – a synthesis of design, function and performance; and
- the environment – internal, external and combined.

For a successful mission, these elements have to be both mutually supportive and properly integrated. The three elements become highly interdependent with variations in one component having a major effect on the others.[1] Within this triptych, experience has shown that the human component is the crucial factor because of a singular capacity for sensory and perceptual discrimination combined with swiftness and accuracy of response to a specific stimulus. Equally, experience has indicated that these human abilities may be compromised by physiological, environmental and psychological factors, as well as spacecraft systems.[2]

It is axiomatic that the manned space flight program has taken a central place in the public's perception of scientific competence and human endeavour. It is, however, important to realise that this accomplishment is built upon an understanding of the basic and intractable laws of physics for launch, orbital flight, rendezvous and return. The engineering accomplishment to meet these goals is evolving, but in each case a solution of proven reliability is provided to meet an absolute requirement. Ground support and crew selection and function are more diffuse. Factors which are recognised to influence crew performance are listed in Table 1. In space flight, crew functions may be divided into sensory, control, processing and memory, together

---

Table 1. Psychological and social factors that influence performance of space crews

Psychological	**Social**
■ limits of performance	■ leadership
■ cognitive abilities	■ crew composition
■ decision-making	■ social skills
■ motivation	
■ attitudes	
■ emotion/moods	
■ psychological stability	
■ personality variables	
■ human reliability (error rate)	
■ productivity	
■ adaptability	
■ time compression	

---

with motor factors. Man's inherent ability to discern patterns, make decisions and plan is superior to the in-built capabilities of existing robotic hardware of comparable cost, weight and size. However, the human senses are inferior in the detection and processing of incoming signals, in detecting small variations in these signals and in response time.[3]

Man is essentially a single channel sequential recorder with a reasonably wide base and low sensitivity input-output capacity in relation to his cost and size.[4] As such, the flexibility of the human response is limited, showing a poor match to the displays and control systems and the operator's mental and physical capabilities. Thus, operator delays are a key area of concern in complex systems. Despite these considerations, man has a distinct advantage over a machine in his capacity to select, ignore, interpret and store many units of information. However, when he is fatigued or under stress, much of this input-output capacity is compromised. In these circumstances, man has a predilection for reverting to a more primitive mode in which he deals with stimuli and responses singly and sequentially so that competing signals must wait for his attention and a defined course of action. Similarly, sleep disturbance may have major effects – malaise and a temporary reduction intelligence quotient predominating[5] – with consequent operational impairment. Work regimes of crew members are structured to avoid undue fatigue and maintain an operable workload.

Certainly established fatigue is associated with clear changes, including:
■ reduction in skill and proficiency;
■ psychological stress;
■ decrements in motivation;
■ decrements in performance; and
■ slow, irregular or distorted performance.

Interestingly, sleep-loss of 60 hours combined with physical inactivity has resulted in decreased insulin sensitivity at peripheral receptor sites and a reduction in the body's ability to handle a glucose load.[6]

In the early years of space flight, a crew member's role was limited to a few tasks and there were doubts about his capabilities. Astronaut performance, however, particularly during emergency or unforeseen events, demonstrated human adaptability and effectiveness. Thus, over time and with the increasing complexity of spacecraft systems, man has evolved from a limited operator to a mission manager, increasingly skilled in information, management and processing.[7] The magnitude of this increase in systems management in the US Space Programme is documented in Table 2.

Table 2. Crew displays and controls in US spacecraft

	Panels	Work Station Elements	Control Display Number/Modes	Computers
Mercury	3	1	143	0
Gemini	7	2	354	1
Apollo	40	7	1,374	4/50
Skylab	189	20	2,980	4
Shuttle	97	9	2,300	5/140
Space Station	200	40	3,000	9/200

As with the evolution and complexity of manned spacecraft systems, so too the functions of the crew are designated into categories of expertise: pilot astronauts and science astronauts. With different requirements and functions in space, the psychological profile of the astronauts differ.[8] These are listed in Tables 3 and 4. Irrespective of these differences, it is essential for all astronauts to be compatible in the confines of a space craft, and a selection, training and support system has evolved

---

Table 3. Psychological characteristics of pilot astronauts (Class 1)

- Military-trained
- Intelligent
- Resilient
- Well-organised
- Pragmatic
- Aggressive/non-hostile
- Ambitious

- Confident, not introspective
- Subtle sense of humour
- Interpersonal relationships in a distant manner
- High motivation:
  - flying
  - mastering increasingly complex systems

Table 4. Psychological characteristics of science astronauts (Classes 2 and 3)

- Intelligent
- Higher scores of verbal/mathematical/engineering achievement
- Spaceflight means to an end
- No driving ambition be in space
- Impatience with routine procedures
- More openly aggressive
- Resolve to complete a task irrespective of merit

---

to enhance and maintain compatibility (Table 5). Thus, an established crew in orbit can determine priorities and risks, recognise targets and opportunities, and improvise in unforeseen circumstances[9] aided by the information available to the crew and ground controllers (Table 6).

Studies have shown[10] that decisions are the result of cognitive information which has the following components:
- prior knowledge of the data source;
- memories of past or similar occurrences;
- simplification rules of heuretics employed by the operator; and
- the operator's inherent bias.

Some of these factors may be modified through training while others are singularly resistant to change.

Table 5. Selective measures which influence crew member's behaviour and performance

Selection
- In-depth selection

Training
- Environmental adaptation
- Social sensitivity
- Team effort
- Cross training
- In-flight maintenance of proficiency
- Self-control

Support
- Work/rest
- Avoiding excessive workload
- Ground contact
- Job rotation
- Recreation
- Exercise
- Recognition awards/benefits

Table 6. Space systems information

	Total Measurements	Displayed to Crew	Displayed to Mission Control
Mercury	100	53	85
Gemini	225	75	202
Apollo Command Module	475	280	336
Apollo Lunar Module	473	214	279
Skylab	2,241	615	2,034
Shuttle	7,831	2,170	3,826
Space Station	10,000	4,000	4,000

Although major decisions have largely been the responsibility of ground support personnel and the link with the ground is fundamental, more sophisticated systems will result in greater crew autonomy. Crew irritability and fatigue have been noticed in relation to in-flight illness, and irritability particularly noticeable when schedules become too demanding.[11] Thus, proper sequencing of tasks is also important, with simple tasks performed efficiently at much higher levels of fatigue than more complex tasks.[12]

It is instructive to consider two major failures in the manned space craft program. The worst was the Challenger explosion in January 1986, with the loss of the orbiter and crew. The prime cause of the explosion after launch was hot gas propellant leaking from an O ring joint on a solid booster after contraction of the joint in an abnormally low ambient air temperature prior to launch.[13] The thorough and open investigation also identified in earlier missions pre-launch pressures on the system and crew which were undesirable. In particular, the factors were:
■ hardware problems;
■ customer requests;
■ operational constraints; and
■ external factors.

The cumulative workload caused is illustrated by Figure 1, suggesting a response by the Centre to accommodate changes from requests that were independently generated, not co-ordinated and that the impact of the cumulative changes was a doubling of workload, impairing the broad oversight of safety and efficiency.

Figure 1

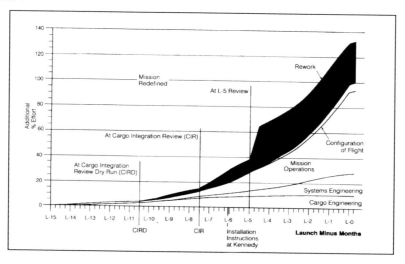

The second major incident was the collision between a Progress supply craft and the Mir space station, resulting in a life-threatening puncture in the station with acute decompression. Until 1977, the Russians used a docking system called Kurs (Course). This automatic system was operated by guidance computers triangulating radar signals from various antennae on the ship and the station. This mapped and executed the complex series of booster firings and breaking that allowed the ships to glide together and effortlessly dock. The system reflected a national philosophy of central control which meant that the docking was not allowed to be in the hands of the cosmonauts. On a number of occasions the Kurs system had been inoperative, resulting in manual dockings.

With these problems in mind, the Russians adopted the Toru system where the commander of Mir sat on a raised seat rather like a stationary bicycle and from a television monitor guided the incoming space craft with joy sticks. Toru was introduced partly because of a shortage of Kurs units and partly because of a change of docking philosophy, the implications of which were not thoroughly considered; in particular, there was a lack of appreciation that the commander guiding the system needed to be mentally fresh and particularly alert. At the time of the accident, Vasily Tsibliyev had been dealing with recurrent problems for weeks on Mir and systematically deprived of sleep prior to the docking which resulted in the decompression, factors which in retrospect point to a decrement of performance and its serious consequences.

In view of the manned space craft philosophy and its undoubted success are there lessons for the assessment of the surgeon, his capabilities at the end of formal training and re-validation of the established practitioner? Just as NASA recognised the centrality of the astronaut, so too the surgeon and his interface with the patient are paramount. Following the NASA parallel, the surgeon should have confidence in the hospital and the medical regulatory system, be technically efficient and accomplished in pre- and post-operative care and rehabilitation, as well as have the humanity and ability to explain the inherent difficulties and dangers to the patient to enable the patient to make an informed choice.

A strong parallel also exists with the interest generated and expressed by the public in both manned space flight activities and in many aspects of medical practice. This may produce special interest groups which are active either locally or nationally or it may produce dogmatic advice from non-medical professional bodies with a declared interest. All are appropriate and heartening but potentially distracting or wrong in philosophy or practical implications. It is unwise to assume that a given discipline or focus group may have the same accomplishment and ability as another and the NASA policy of being open to ideas but willing to challenge and demand proof of validity should be adopted. It may be that a more robust attitude towards challenging outside advice has been a recent failing of the medical profession.

A cardinal feature of current Western surgical attitude is unease with a central regulatory body, either a government body or an institutional healthcare provider which are perceived to be remote, bureaucratic and unsympathetic to the needs of the surgeon. This results in a background of remote regulation.

Taking the UK as an example, recent years have seen the introduction of the hospital Trust system, European Union directives (Calman) training, a research and development funding scheme (Culyer), major changes in the philosophy and training of nurses, regulation and assessment of university departments' research and teaching assessments, and a proliferation of bureaucratic mechanisms to support these activities. All derived from different sources and committees in an uncoordinated manner, adding considerably to the workload of the consultant surgeon who was already working at least one-third above contractual requirements.[14] Similarly in the US, a divide has developed between the private insurer offering a diversity of insurance choices but using up to 25% of each health dollar in administrative overheads and potentially not delivering comprehensive healthcare. It is arguable that the estrangement of the surgeon from the central regulatory and funding authority departs from the NASA model of selective support and enhancement of performance. In addition, the advent of diffuse extensive and uncoordinated changes with unpredictable interactions affecting the surgical environment could be regarded as a phenomenon described in Figure 1 as 'an identified undesirable scenario leading to confusion and inefficiency together with the decrement of performance'.

The technical aspects of surgical skill are amenable to simulator reproduction. NASA crew selection profiles suggest some personal characteristics are more responsive to assessment than others. Essentially the assessment is a mechanism of instruction and a check of competence for the flight deck crew — the pilot astronaut. A comparison of the characteristics listed in Tables 3 and 4 suggest that some of the traits desirable in a surgeon may be more prevalent in the science astronaut who is potentially more resistant to repetitive outside supervision. However, the surgeon may also possess the virtues of cognitive thought and adaptability which may manifest with increasing seniority and the combination of such characteristics is the essential basis of a good surgeon.

A course in anaesthetic crisis resource management analogous to courses in crew cockpit resource management conducted in military and commercial aviation has been developed.[15, 16] The anaesthetist received didactic instruction in dynamic decision-making in a familiar institution dealing with acute cardiovascular, pulmonary, metabolic, neurological and equipment emergencies. Scores on written tests of knowledge showed significant improvement for trainees but not for established senior staff, suggesting that established practitioners may achieve a plateau of performance in repetitive practical skills which may be identified in clinical outcome.

Assessment of a surgeon will encompass two principal aspects, technical expertise and pre- and post-operative care. Compared to manned space flight competence, surgical competence may be more difficult to assess. Technical skills certainly may be tested using a simulator and for manipulative procedures may have true value. However, considering the totality of surgical care, a simulator could prove to be of less value. Certainly simulation is of proven value in manned space flight as it tests response to absolutes, which may not be the case in clinical practice. A possible example of divergence is in the simulation and management of shock. In the clinical setting, it may be difficult to recognise the components of hypovolemic and septic shock which may co-exist and the failure to do so at the bedside will result in a simulation exercise which may not be entirely appropriate. In addition, the pathogenesis of shock is not fully elucidated and no absolute reproduction of the mechanism is therefore possible – it is only 12 years since it was demonstrated that vascular endothelial cells are able to generate nitric oxide gas.[15, 16] The nitric oxide produced influences the degree of vasodilation by passing from endothelial to smooth muscle cells to active soluble guanylate cyclase and by so doing produces vascular relaxation, and inhibits platelet aggregation and vascular smooth muscle proliferation. Yet in a simulation of endotoxic shock are the actions of this powerful substance factored in or, indeed, can they be, with the patho-physiological role only partly understood and the capacity of the individual patient to synthesize nitric oxide complex and obscure?

Yet another developing study is the role of adrenomedullin in disease. Adrenomedullin is another hypotensive peptide originally isolated from human phaeochromocytoma[17] and adrenomedullin mRNA is strongly expressed in vascular endothelium, vascular smooth muscle cells and human lung tissue. It decreases pulmonary vascular resistance in a dose-dependent manner with plasma levels elevated in pulmonary hypotension, congenital cyanotic heart disease and hypoxaemia due to lung disease. These observations raise the possibility that adrenomedullin is involved in the physiology of pulmonary circulation and in the pathophysiology of hypoxaemia but its exact role remains obscure. In consequence, an appropriate simulation is not directly applicable and does not directly relate to a NASA simulation model following absolute values and laws.

This is not to dismiss simulation as it does offer scenarios which may be of benefit by:
- simulating critical events at no risk to the patient;
- reproducing a specific critical event repetitively;
- providing an opportunity to halt simulation for discussion and teaching;
- allowing errors to be made and their consequences explained;
- providing a record and critique of performance;
- allowing objective evaluation of performance;
- allowing uncommon events to be experienced; and
- allowing control of independent or multiple variables.

Thus, technical aspects of surgery may benefit greatly from simulation for both assessment of competence and evidence of retention of expertise, but other fundamental aspects of surgical patient management may only be modelled approximately.

At NASA, astronauts are periodically assessed but is this feasible for surgeons? And can costs be contained? A proposal would be intermittent selective assessment of established practitioners, and mandatory assessment of trainees at the end of the prescribed period of training. A possible method of selective assessment would be a study of the mortality and morbidity rates for a given individual which could be identified as outside of a yet-to-be defined acceptable range. Such a limited system would need to be initiated by looking at outcome.

Irvin and Wallace[18] looked at 308 patients with colorectal cancer treated between 1991 and 1995 with data collected simultaneously by three sources – the hospital management, junior surgical staff and a personal audit held by the consultant. The junior data did not record 35% of patients and 67 post-operative complications, did not provide data of recurrence of the disease, together with a lower five-year survival rate of 29 +/- 7.4% compared to the consultant audit figure of 45 +/- 7.1%. The computerised data held by the hospital management missed 50 post-operative complications and provided no information on local recurrence of the rectal cancers. Thus, outcome, even if reliably recorded, may be determined by factors outside the surgeon's direct control and the collection of valid and agreed data will be fundamental.

In a recent study of the outcome of treatment of patients with colorectal cancer, age, tumour stage and differentiation and mode of admission were regarded as significant independent prognostic variables.[19] After adjustment for these variables, neither the seniority of the operating surgeon, the consultant workload nor hospital throughput were identified as factors influencing patient's survival. Similarly, Kee *et al* [20] studied the mortality after 54 months of 3,217 new patients with colorectal cancer registered over four years. Strong predictors of survival were Duke's stage, tumour differentiation and distant spread, as well as whether or not the patient presented as an emergency admission. Thus, retrospective data collection assessment is fraught and may actually deceive. It remains uncertain how practical and expensive a robust and verifiable system may prove to be, but certainly current methods are not reliable.

There are some clear parallels with NASA crew selection policy. The criteria for the ideal surgeon identified by The Royal College of Surgeons (Table 7) shows a marked similarity to the NASA flight crew criteria and although both may reflect simply a cherished ideal, there is accumulated evidence that the NASA criteria have proven effective. Assuming the ideal has been attained, how can the surgeon's function be monitored? The patient selection for assessment of competence in general surgery should ideally reflect the prevalence of conditions presenting to a general surgeon as part of his workload (Table 8) as described by Allen-Mersh and Earlam.[21] Selection of the predominant case-mix would at least provide a clinical basis for assessment of competence or re-evalidation relating to present day common clinical practice; the second strand should be assessment in the surgeon's declared sub-speciality.

Table 7. Desirable skills for a surgical trainee

■ Communication skills	■ Surgical skills and manual dexterity
■ Knowledge of basic sciences	■ Post-operative management
■ Knowledge of theoretical clinical skills	■ Teaching and learning skills
■ Knowledge of clinical skills	■ Management and leadership skills
■ Decision making – treatment options	■ Research and data analysis skills

---

Table 8. Incidence of general surgical operations

Incidence of general surgical operations	Number per 100,000 of population
Appendicectomy	143.5
Inguinal hernia repair	129.6
Benign breast disease	75.5
Cholecystectomy	73.9
Anal surgery	71.6
Cystoscopy	62.3
Varicose veins	54.7
Malignant skin lesions	51.6
Circumcision	44.6
Mastectomy	29.9
Orchidopexy	23.6
Colectomy	21.2
Rectal carcinoma	18.8
Thyroidectomy	17.3
Hydrocele	11.7
Femoral hernia repair	11.6
Amputation for vascular disease	8.7
Defunctioning colostomy	8.0

A system exists for the assessment of the competence of trainees and their ability to sustain independent clinical practice. However, the introduction of re-validation for established practitioners, a system which is not of clear value where it has been discussed, raises the bizarre possibility of one-half of the profession being actively involved in assessing the other half to the ultimate detriment of clinical services with high-cost overheads.

At NASA flight operations, the mission is planned and executed on the basis of an agreed mission plan, with identification of problems and potential solutions, together with training for crew training in flexibility to meet the unexpected. Similarly, surgery is to the patient a monumental event causing great anxiety and ideally a successful, but potentially uncertain, outcome. The real skill in the NASA model is the identification, anticipation and correction of difficulties before they occur. The clinical parallel would be the identification of potential complications across the whole spectrum of care: pre-operative risk factors, reduced technical competence, the management of post-operative complications and problems of rehabilitation. There may be some evidence that this approach improves clinical outcome.[22] A clinical assessment based upon predicted management has, like space flight, a discernible outcome.

Recent work[23] has utilised the physiological and operative severity score for the enumeration of mortality and morbidity (Possum) to give an estimation of the risk of complications and death after surgery. The Physiological and Operative Severity Score for Enumeration of Mortality and Morbidity (Possum) has been developed from the multi-variate discriminate analysis of factors measured in a broad group of surgical patients. Using commonly recorded parameters the system determines a Physiological Score and an Operative Severity Score from which expected morbidity and mortality rates can be calculated using logistic regression equations. The further refinement of the methodology, P-Possum, has, for vascular surgery patients, resulted in a prediction not significantly different from the observed death rate. In addition, the system takes into account case-mix, tertiary referral and high-risk patients. Use of a Possum model offers the real possibility that a closer assessment of the individual surgeon's performance to predicted reality may be possible. This may have the function of a screening system for identifying individuals who potentially underachieve. The application of the NASA flight model for surgeons identified by the Possum system would be a pre-operative patient assessment and management plan for the prospective management of a given patient. Diseases which are common within the discipline and declared sub-speciality may thus be assessed with a clear clinical mechanism for management and definable end outcome.

A space flight to an astronaut presents a challenge, causing fear, exhilaration and satisfaction with a successful outcome. The centrality of the system is the astronaut and the spacecraft systems. Similarly, the relationship between the surgeon and the patient is at the heart of clinical practice. In both, the emotions associated with such major events are almost identical. Learning from the outstanding success of the manned spacecraft system, practitioner competence is ideally prospectively assessed, and the practitioner should be content that the system is providing proper support, is open to suggestions for improvement and will change if assessed as valid. With evidence that astronaut performance may be degraded by fatigue, it is essential that the surgeon should be properly rested, and that he is in control of the local environment in order to produce proper support for the centrality of clinical practice, namely the essentially confidential doctor-patient interaction.

If a surgeon is identified as a poor performer, it has been suggested that respected senior members of specialist surgical societies should be available to assist in solving the problem.[24] Ideally their role should be supportive and comprise responsible investigation with suggestions for extra training. The specialist society through a regulatory body, such as The Royal College of Surgeons, should provide this training on a national basis. Whatever the established mechanism, a system of prospective evaluation has been proven over decades at NASA and is worthy of consideration for terrestrial use.

References

1. Nicogossian AE. Human factors for Mars missions. In: Rather DB, ed. *NASA Mars Conference* Vol 71. American Aeronautical Society; 1988.

2. Christensen JM, Talbot JM. *Research Opportunities in Human Behaviour and Performance NASA CR-3886.* Washington, DC: National Aeronautics and Space Administration, Scientific and Technical Information Branch; 1985.

3. Wargo MJ, Kelly CR, Mitchell MB, Prosin DJ. *Human Operator Response, Speed, Frequency and Flexibility NASA CR-874.* Washington, DC: National Aeronautics and Space Administration; September 1987.

4. Hartman BO. Psychological aspects of aerospace medicine. In: Randel HW, ed. *Aerospace Medicine.* 2nd ed. Baltimore: Williams and Wilkins; 1971.

5. Colquhoun WP. Circadian variations in mental efficiency. In: *Biological Rhythm and Human Performance.* Academic Press; 1971. pp39-107.

6. Van Helder T, Symonds JD, Radomski MW. Effects of sleep deprivation and exercise on glucose tolerance. *Aviation Space and Environmental Medicine* 1993; 64:487-492.

7. Loftus JP. Evolution of the astronaut's role. In: Montemerio MD and Crow AC, ed. Workshop Proceedings -- *Space Human Factors Vol 1.* Washington, DC: National Aeronauts and Space Administration; 1982.

8. Harding R. Selection and training. In: *Survival in Space.* London and New York: Routledge; 1989. pp137-143.

9.   Beoczy AK. Distribution of man-machine controls in space teleoperations. In: *Proceedings of the Behaviour Objectives in Aviation Automated Systems Symposium.* 1982, 114.

10.   Markes TE, Howell WC. Intuitive Frequency Judgements as a Function of Prior Expectations. *Observed Evidence and Individual Processing Strategies (Technical Report 79-06).* Rice University, Decer.

11.   Cooper HSF. *A House in Space.* Bantam Books; 1976.

12.   Welford AT. *Fundamentals of Skill.* London: Methuen and Co; 1968.

13.   *Report of the Presidential Commission on the Space Shuttle Challenger Accident.* US Government Printing Service; 1986. pp164-177.

14.   The Association of Surgeons of Great Britain and Ireland. *Report of a Confidential Enquiry into Hours Worked and Private Practice Remuneration.* London; 1994.

15.   Palmer RM, Ferrige AG, Moncada S. Nitric oxide release accounts for the biological activity of endothelium-derived releasing factor. *Nature* 1987; 327:524-526.

16.   Howard SK, Gaba DM, Fuh KJ, Yang S, Sannquist FH. Anaesthetic crisis resource management training: Teaching anaesthesiologists to handle critical incidents. *Aviation Space and Environmental Medicine* 1992; 63:763-770.

17.   Kitamura K, Kangawa K, Kawamojo M. Adrenomedullin: A novel Hypotensive peptide isolated from human phaeochromocytoma. *Biochemical and Biophysical Research Communications* 1993; 192:553-560.

18.   Irvin TT, Wallace J. Auditing clinical performance – what statistics do we believe? *British Journal of Surgery* 1999; 86:Supplement 1:83.

19.   Parry JM, Collins S, Mathews J, Scott NA, Woodman CBJ. Influence of volume of work on the outcome of treatment for patients with colorectal cancer. *British Journal of Surgery* 1999;86:475-481.

20.   Kee F, Wilson RH, Harper C, Patterson CC, McCallion K, Horston RF, Moorhead RJ, Sloan JM, Newlands BJ. Influence of hospital and clinical workload on survival from colorectal cancer: Cohort study. *British Medical Journal* 1999; 318:1381-1385.

21.   Allen-Mersh TG, Earlam RJ. General surgical workload in England and Wales. *British Medical Journal* 1983; 287:1115-1118.

22.   Wilson J, Woods I, Fawcett J, Whall R, Dibb W, Morris C, McManus E. Reducing the risk of major elective surgery: Randomised controlled trial of pre-operative optimisation of oxygen delivery. *British Medical Journal* 1999; 318:1099-1103.

23.   Midwinter MJ, Tytherleigh M, Ashley S. Estimation of mortality and morbidity risk in vascular surgery using Possum and the Portsmouth Predictor Equation. *British Journal of Surgery* 1999; 86:471-474.

24.   Humphreys WV. Audit of the surgeon: Problems and perspectives. *British Journal of Surgery* 1998; 85:1167-1170.

The Opportunities for Virtual Reality & Simulation in the Training and Assessment of Technical Surgical Skills

R J Stone BSc (Hons), MSc, CPsychol, AFBPsS, MErgS, Eur Erg, FIoN, FVRS

Virtual Presence Limited (Manchester & London) and
North of England Wolfson Centre for Minimally Invasive Therapy

Abstract

The prohibitive costs and technological difficulties of implementing surgical simulators based on comprehensive virtual humans using dynamic visual, tactile, auditory and even olfactory data have prompted a number of computer-based training (CBT) proponents to carry out a radical rethink of their methodological approaches. One example, MIST (Minimally Invasive Surgical Trainer) evolved from a comprehensive in-theatre task analysis, based on sound ergonomics principles, to ensure that the final product actually measures what its original development team intended it to measure. MIST is a British PC-based 'keyhole' surgical trainer which uses commercial virtual reality (VR) and database software to foster and document trainees' acquisition of minimally invasive surgery skills, thereby enhancing skills assessment during initial training and career revalidation points. This paper puts MIST developments into the context of worldwide developments in VR generally (hardware, software and surgical applications) and addresses some of the key issues to bear in mind when considering CBT as a solution to medical training and assessment.

INTRODUCTION

Over the past two years and, after an incubation period lasting some six to seven years, the field of endeavour popularly referred to as virtual reality (VR) has experienced something of a revival, a revival that has taken the form of a number of important developments which have helped VR to become an accessible, usable and justifiable member of the computer-based training (CBT) fraternity for many applications, particularly in the arena of medical and surgical training.

But what exactly has changed? VR, in its attempt to promote intuitive, real-time interaction with three-dimensional databases,[1] has evolved from a purely (and quite limited) visual interactive experience to become a mature toolkit for which there are, today, real applications and evidence of financial, training and assessment benefits. Preoccupation with the once-ubiquitous head-mounted display (HMD) and so-called immersive VR has diminished, for the time being at least. Desktop implementations (using standard computer screens), together with conventional or stereoscopic image projection systems have become popular in recent years. 'Higher-end' visualisation techniques, such as the CAVE (small rooms defined by large video projection walls) and dome-based or 'wrap-around' imaging systems are highly impressive. However, in the medical world, they tend to be restricted to wealthy foundation or governmental research laboratories and not focused on real-world cost-effective applications.

The most important change has been the arrival of low-cost, industry-standard multimedia computers and high-performance graphics hardware. Coupled with this, the spread of VR modelling and run-time software (eg DirectX, OpenGL, VRML, panoramic digital imaging tools, even some PC games engines), together with low-cost and free resources from the Web, is beginning to make VR much more accessible to the non-specialist user or developer than was the case just two years ago.

VR AND THE MEDICAL COMMUNITY

During the late 1980s, many visionaries – notably at the University of North Carolina and within the Department of Defence in the US – were developing the notion of the surgeon or consultant of the future, equipped with a head-mounted display and rehearsing procedures in VR from detailed inspections of an unborn foetus, through to the accurate targeting of energy in radiation therapy, even socket fit testing in total joint replacement. For many years, the US led the field in medical VR, and some of the early conferences and exhibitions delivered many promises about how technology would revolutionise surgery in the new millennium. Many of those promises would, even today, be hard-pushed to reach reality before 2050, let alone 2000.

Nevertheless, in 1995, one of the leading practical advocates of virtual environments in the US, Colonel Richard Satava, attempted to categorise achievable applications of VR in medical and surgical domains.[2] He saw developments in the fields of surgical intervention and planning, medical therapy, preventative medicine, medical training and skill enhancement, database visualisation and much more. Satava's original work, sponsored by the Advanced Research Projects Agency, ARPA, focused on large-scale robotic or telepresence surgery systems, using VR technologies to recreate the sense of presence for a distant surgeon when operating on, say, a battlefield casualty. However, other research efforts began to emerge across the States (and Europe) using VR in a classic simulator mode to rehearse or plan delicate operations (eg total joint replacement or in certain ophthalmic operations). It was then shown that one could actually use the successful virtual procedures to back up *in situ* performance (ie through the projection of 3-D graphics onto the operative site – 'augmented reality').

Other programs saw the future not as either robot or surgeon, but as a combination of the two with the automated component of the operating theatre augmenting the skill of the surgeon, having been thoroughly pre-programd in a pre-operative virtual world.[3] Augmented reality took a step further when, as early as 1993, a magnetic resonance image (MRI) had been taken of a patient and overlaid onto a real-time video image of the head.[4]

During the late 1980s and early 1990s, the application of VR and associated technologies to the field of medicine and surgery steadily increased, with pioneering companies such as High Techsplanations (HT Medical) and CinÈmed becoming responsible for fuelling the obsession with 'making surgical simulation real'.[5] However, very recent conferences and exhibitions suggest a plateau may have been reached, with some of the front-running concepts undergoing a period of consolidation through clinical validation. Tried and tested products, available at prices that are affordable to the greater majority of surgical teaching institutions, are still somewhat elusive. Nevertheless, the key uses of VR remain as Satava predicted, with many projects receiving academic grant support or national and continental funding (as one finds in Europe, with the Framework V Initiative, for example).

Developments in technology continue to deliver more and more robust hardware and software and the surgical community gradually becomes more and more involved (albeit at a snail's pace in the UK, it sometimes seems, with collaboration between currently fragmented groups still desperately needed to avoid wasteful reproduction of effort).

A paper such as this cannot hope to cover all historical and contemporary aspects of VR and medicine/surgery under a single cover. However the interested reader can obtain a more in-depth appreciation by accessing the Web pages provided at the end of the text[6,7] and by selectively reading papers in the excellent publications of Westwood *et al.*[8,9]

'TECHNOLOGY PUSH'

Despite the coming of the PC/Windows era, bringing with it the capability of delivering highly interactive virtual medical environments (attractive to resource-limited surgical teaching bodies), the international academic research community (in the main) still shows a bias towards sophisticated anatomical and physiological simulations of the human body, hosted on graphics supercomputers. From the digital reconstruction of microtomed bodies of executed convicts (eg the Visible Human Project[10]) to speculative deformable models of various organs and vascular systems (eg Forschungszentrum Karlsruhe[11] and University of California Berkeley's VESTA project – Virtual Environments for Surgical Training and Augmentation[12]), the quest to deliver comprehensive 'virtual humans' using dynamic visual, tactile, auditory and even olfactory modes of interaction looks set to continue into the foreseeable future. The problem is: who in the real surgical world can afford to procure, operate and maintain such systems? Do they really offer trainee and consultant surgeons a career-enhancing advantage?

One can attribute the failure to deliver practical and affordable training and assessment systems based on VR partly to a lack of technological appreciation and experience on the part of individual surgical specialists or administrators within the research organisations concerned. In the recent past, a good number of institutions have purchased VR equipment, often on the basis of what looks to be an attractive discount or with promises of free technical support. However, it has soon been discovered that owning a VR system is not as straightforward as it might seem, for at least two reasons.

First, the development of bespoke, high fidelity libraries of correctly behaving virtual anatomical and physiological datasets is extremely complex. Such libraries do not exist as ready-to-use, off-the-shelf products and the in-house resources required to produce such datasets can be enormous. As will be discussed below, many VR technologies have not yet developed to a level where they can be used to provide meaningful and experimentally reliable data on surgical performance. A wrist-mounted electromagnetic tracking system may, if correctly set up, provide reasonable data on the spatial motion of the wrist, but will not provide an overall metric of arm-wrist-hand-digit dexterity.

Secondly, the poor uptake also stems from an equally poor understanding – sometimes on the part of the original simulation developers – the medical needs and ergonomic requirements of the surgical users and trainees. Furthermore, it is all too often easy to forget that most medical organisations simply cannot justify the excessive initial costs of so-called graphics 'supercomputers' – not to mention crippling annual maintenance charges, depreciation and, in today's rapidly changing IT world, rapid technological redundancy.

VR PERIPHERAL TECHNOLOGIES

VR has stimulated the emergence of an impressive range of new and, in many cases, reasonably cheap computer interface technologies. Many of these 'peripherals' – devices operated or worn by the human user in order to input data into the computer – never end up as de facto components of turn-key VR systems. They tend to appear instead as repackaged 'high-tech' solutions to long-standing problems in the assessment of human-computer interfaces, or as attempts to quantify certain features of psychomotor skill.

For example, in the mid-1990s, the company Ingersoll-Rand adapted a commercially available VR hand exoskeletal device called the Dextrous Hand Master (developed by the US company Exos Inc) by endowing the physical structure of the multi-link device with resistive ink force sensors. The Ergo Quantifier, as it was known, was designed primarily for evaluating the effects of equipment design on the performance of the human hand, but was advertised as a keyboard ergonomics analysis tool to assess the potential risk of repetitive strain injury based on individual typing styles. Although the Ergo Quantifier was delivered as a PC-based solution with its own suite of software, it faded into oblivion quite rapidly. It is likely that the product's demise was caused by technical and reliability problems with the DHM system (which was one of the better peripheral VR devices at the time), coupled with the dexterity restrictions it imposed upon its wearers (thereby introducing artefacts into keystroke analyses).

This is but one example which stresses caution when considering the use of technology – VR or otherwise – for assessing human skill. Today, it is possible to purchase a wide range of devices – multi-axis controllers, instrumented gloves, haptic feedback joysticks, electromagnetic trackers, physiological monitoring units for 'biocontrol' (eg low-cost EEG, EMG, EOG), 'wearable computers' with monocular and binocular headsets, and so on. Each class of device has its own merits and limitations, with the latter rarely being made explicit on marketing or technical support material. However, there is one important fact to bear in mind: VR peripheral technologies are not precision scientific instruments. Nevertheless, in the right hands, the potential for using these imprecise products to solve certain conventional ergonomic and interface issues is considerable.

WHAT CAN VR DELIVER BESIDES SENSORY EXPERIENCES?

It is not just the peripheral technologies from VR markets which, when in the right hands, can contribute to the assessment of human performance. The very object-oriented nature of many current VR run-time and data management packages make them ideal application programming environments for recording – even replaying – the user's performance when navigating and interacting within a virtual environment. Consequently, recent efforts by a small number of international institutions and companies have focused on adding value to their simulations by endowing otherwise 'dumb' virtual environments and objects with an ability to record user-induced motions, handling times, collisions (both intentional and erroneous), and so on. One example of such a system will be described later. But what, returning to the topic of surgical assessment, should VR systems actually record?

Darzi *et al* claim that 'finding objective criteria for judging good surgical technique is difficult'.[13] In fact, the problem is much more acute than this and one should, perhaps, replace the word 'good' with 'any'. However, from an assessment standpoint, specialists from the ergonomics community will contest the claim that it is difficult to find objective criteria in the assessment of all skill-based activities. Indeed, the disciplines of ergonomics and applied psychology have, for the latter half of the 20th century, made significant advances in developing techniques for the analysis of tasks characterised by specialist decision-making and psychomotor behaviours.[14] Some of the techniques for measuring such features as mental workload or mental resource, cognitive performance, perceptual-motor skills and situational awareness have been subjected to quite stringent validation, when integrated within appropriate experimental designs and regimes.[15,16,17,18,19] However, a good many still rely on quite antiquated products and, when exposed to users in a contemporary setting, require considerable subjective effort on the part of the administrator during the interpretation of results.

Virtual reality, coupled with a competently programd database management system, offers the means by which subjectivity in performance assessment can be significantly reduced, even removed altogether. However, this statement is only true if the VR system, or the peripheral technology used, is selected and implemented so that it measures what the researcher intended it to measure. This is typically referred to as the ecological validity of an instrument or experimental design. It is generally agreed that the term competency refers to an individual's knowledge, skills or abilities (sometimes called 'KSAs') performed to an acceptable standard when observed or recorded in the individual's place of work. It should – stress should – make little or no difference if that place of work is real or virtual.

WHAT IS BEING MEASURED?

The Importance of an Ergonomics Task Analysis

'Attention comes first, learning after attention is focused. And learning is primarily action...' (Dewey *et al*, in Bricken[20]).

'The most important principle of classroom activity design is that the students' actions determine what will be learned...' (Walker, in Bricken[20]).

The most important three words in these quotes are attention, action and learning. By its very nature, VR is an attention-grabbing medium with the anecdotal intrinsic motivational qualities such a feature commands (ie learning or information retention are improved and subsequent performance in the real world equivalent is enhanced). Increasingly, the VR community is providing good examples, with objective measures, of transfer of training – improved performance (eg faster learning rates and fewer errors) in the real world following training in the virtual world equivalent. This is a key issue for the medical community and one that will accelerate the uptake of VR once valid and reliable results from the growing installed base of experimental simulator prototypes are published in reputable journals.

However, to achieve this, one has, once again, to turn to the ergonomics and applied psychology community, not just for guidance in the appropriate design of experimental programs[15,16,17] but for guidance in the structured analysis of real-world surgical tasks. Additionally, one needs to be able to use the results of such an analysis to specify the abstraction of the real-world task elements into their VR counterparts.

An excellent definition of task analysis was put forward by Bradley of axsWave Software, Inc, based on two IBM documents compiled by Terrio & Vreeland[21] and Snyder.[22] A task analysis is an ordered sequence of tasks and subtasks, which identifies the performer or user; the action, activities or operations; the environment; the starting state; the goal state; and the requirements to complete a task such as hardware, software or information.

Without a properly executed task analysis, one runs the risk of specifying or designing a VR (or any CBT or multimedia) system that fails to record or measure those elements of human skill one was targeting in the first place. One also jeopardises the future integrity of any experimental program that sets out to validate one's training and assessment concept, not to mention the transfer of training from the virtual to the real.

An example: MIST (Minimally Invasive Surgical Trainer)

During the second half of 1994 and early in 1995, numerous articles appeared in the British press and on mainstream TV news programs which cast serious doubt on the future of 'keyhole' surgery, specifically those practices in support of laparoscopic cholecystectomy. The fact that patients had died or had been left in considerable pain, sometimes as a result of surgeon error, led to serious calls for action, especially with regard to improving the training and assessment of surgeons 'graduating' from conventional, open surgery, onto these more remote techniques. In the UK, unlike the US or some countries within continental Europe, live animal-based training is prohibited. As a result, primary laparoscopic experience is typically fostered through the remote handling of sweets or candy, grapes, raw chicken tissue, plastic tubing, foam-mounted balloons or synthetic body models with replaceable (and, thus, quite costly) organs. This situation, coupled with increasing UK regulatory and certification pressures (the pressures are still evident today), meant that in 1994 the provision of a simulator – with some form of basic, yet integrated means of assessment – was seen as instrumental to the development of specific surgical skills.

Established in the spring of 1994, the North of England Wolfson Centre for Minimally Invasive Therapy commenced operations under grant support from the UK Wolfson Foundation and the British government's Department of Health. Today, as in 1994, the Manchester Centre revolves around a collaborative arrangement between Virtual Presence and Manchester Royal Infirmary (MRI). The collaborators were, over a two-year period, tasked with evaluating VR and related technologies, possibly progressing to a stage whereby a prototype British laparoscopic cholecystectomy simulator could be developed to a state where clinical and human factor evaluations could take place.[23]

User requirements: in-theatre task analyses

The first stage of the Wolfson Centre project involved a number of short in-theatre observation and recording sessions (assisted by specialists at the MRI), using video and digital endoscopy. The aim of these task analyses, which were based on similar exercises carried out by the author, albeit in the applications fields of subsea robotics and the food industry,[24,25] was to obtain a clear understanding of the performance and ergonomic features of the surgeon's task and workplace, addressing such issues as how dexterity and psychomotor skills are affected by:

■ workspace layout;

■ proximity of surgical team (ie how the surgeon's performance is constrained by the physical presence of colleagues and their associated equipment);

■ surgeon's posture (including the need to change and hold postures for certain activities; such as diathermy, the short-term impact of upper-torso fatigue);

■ individual working styles;

■ patient condition; and

■ surgical progress, contingency measures (ie deviations from the 'norm' brought about by sudden changes in patient's state or even surgical errors).

However, another part of the in-theatre exercise involved the evaluation of a number of different forms of media for image capture (and subsequent digitising for the anticipated anatomical texture mapping exercises). In other words, the decision to 'make surgical simulation real'[5] had already been taken. In addition, MRI surgeons provided practical demonstrations of current training practice as well as strictly supervised 'hands-on' experience in order to appreciate the physical properties of human anatomy, such as form, mass, compliance and the extent of movement of the laparoscopic instruments. These exercises, together with lengthy briefing sessions from practising and trainee surgeons, produced a number of conclusions which were very much examples of 'technology push', as criticised earlier. Concerns about how to avoid the use of head-mounted displays but still deliver a 3-D image to the surgeon's eyes (eg via autostereoscopic systems) was but one example of this preoccupation with VR technology. Other areas of recommendation addressed the problems of modelling the deformation of complex virtual tissues and fluid behaviours, or the design of sophisticated haptic interface devices.

Unfortunately, these recommendations served to drive the Wolfson Centre research program forward for at least 12 out of the allocated 24 months. This is not to criticise the work that was actually done, the results of which actually resulted in impressive prototype British systems long before the emergence of their American or Japanese counterparts.[23] However, what was unfortunate was that the real ergonomic findings of the in-theatre task analyses had been ignored, resulting in a research program which, had there not been a radical rethink, would have delivered a simulator which could neither be used nor afforded by most medical teaching institutions.

MIST

The specific result of taking a step back and revisiting the earlier task analyses with a more unbiased approach was the identification of an urgent need to develop a low-cost, PC-based laparoscopic cholecystectomy simulator. What the task analyses had actually produced was a structured decomposition of a range of minimally invasive tasks which could be defined in the form of 'human performance primitives'. It was found that each primitive could be implemented reasonably easily within a proprietary VR software package and each could be endowed with 'academic credibility', particularly from the domains of applied/experimental psychology and human factors (eg Boff & Lincoln[26]).

The end product of these further analyses was MIST, a surgical psychomotor skills trainer based on a commercially available instrumented laparoscopic interface connected to an industry standard PC. Movements from the laparoscopic interface tools (recently redesigned by Virtual Presence and Immersion Corporation) are translated into 3-D computer graphics which accurately track and represent the movements of those tools within a virtual 'operating' volume. Within this volume, simple geometric shapes are generated and subsequently manipulated using the interface tools. The graphics have been intentionally kept simple in order that high frame rates may be maintained on relatively low cost equipment and to preserve the validity and reliability of the simulations when used in applied experimental research.

MIST features five general modes of operation: tutorial, training, examination, analysis and configuration. Closer analysis of the video records generated during the earlier in-theatre observation sessions, together with iterative review sessions involving consultant surgeons and senior registrars, subsequently drove the specification of six basic task modules for MIST, including combinations of instrument approach, target acquisition, target manipulation and placement, transfer between instruments, target contact with optional diathermy, and controlled instrument withdrawal/replacement.

These tasks, described in more detail below, can be configured for varying degrees of difficulty and the configurations saved to a library for re-use. Specific task configurations can be assigned to individual students. In the examination mode the supervisor can select the tasks and repetitions and is able to order and save to a specific file for that trainee. Progress can be assessed with optional performance playback of the training session or examination. Data analyses permit quantification of overall task performance (accuracy and errors, plus sub-task time, time to completion and motion efficiency are logged during the tasks) and right-/left-hand performances. The data are accessible in forms suitable for statistical analysis and significance testing.

The MIST task set

The main interface to MIST is quite simple. As well as the task set-up, calibration and help/text sections, the majority of the display is occupied by the interactive graphics window. In essence, this takes the form of a wire-frame box which describes the effective operating volume in which target stimuli appear, are acquired and can be manipulated by virtual representations of the laparoscopic instruments.

For all tasks, a MIST training session starts when the subject manipulates the instruments to 'touch' a simple start box located in the centre of the operating volume. Once objects have been acquired, successful and erroneous acquisitions are colour-coded appropriately (and recorded).

Task 1: Simple object acquisition and placement

Task 1 tests the subject's ability to acquire an object with either hand and move it to a new 3-D location within the virtual operating volume. The task has relevance to such operative activities as clip placement, tissue removal and gall stone recovery. The system generates a spherical target object at a random position within the operating volume. The subject moves the instrument tip to acquire the sphere. Once acquired, a small wire-frame box appears at a random position within the operating volume and the subject is required to position the sphere within the box. The task is repeated for a set number of repetitions.

Task 2: Between-instrument transfer

Task 2 relates to a fundamental surgical requirement — the transfer of an object from one instrument to another. The task has relevance (for example) to the fundus of the gall bladder being passed between two grasping forceps before being retracted. A more advanced skill application would be passing a needle between two needle holders during suturing. The system generates a spherical target object at a random position within the operating volume. The subject moves the instrument tip to acquire the sphere. Once acquired, the subject is required to pass the sphere to the other instrument. Intersections with the sphere and parts of the instrument other than the tool tips result in deductions to the accuracy score. On successful transfer, a wire-frame box appears at a random position within the operating volume and the subject is required to position the sphere within the box. The task is repeated for a set number of repetitions.

Task 3: Target traversal

Task 3 focuses on sequential instrument-to-instrument transfer — the 'walking' of instruments along vessels or structures to reach their extremities (eg the neck of the gall bladder, as seen at the start of a laparoscopic cholecystectomy). This task in effect combines the skills of Task 1 with Task 2. The system generates a cylindrical target object at a random position within the operating volume. The cylinder is subdivided into a number of segments. The subject is required to grasp the top segment with either instrument, followed by the next segment along the cylinder with the remaining instrument. The procedure is repeated in a step-by-step fashion, alternating between instruments until all segments have been acquired. The task is repeated for a set number of repetitions.

Task 4: Tool withdrawal and insertion

Changing from one instrument type to another and being able to reinsert the new instrument quickly and accurately is a key skill in laparoscopic surgery. In Task 4, the system generates a spherical target object at a random position within the operating volume. The subject moves the instrument tip to acquire the sphere. Once acquired, the remaining instrument is brought into contact with the sphere. After contact has been made, it is then withdrawn completely from the operating volume. The same instrument is then reintroduced to make contact with the sphere. Unintentional collisions with the sphere and other instrument result in deductions to the accuracy score. The task is repeated for a set number of repetitions.

Task 5: Diathermy procedures

Task 5 focuses on the accurate application of diathermy to specific bleeding points in the gall bladder bed. The task requires accurate 3-D location with activation of the diathermy instrument only when appropriate contact has been achieved. The system generates a spherical target object at a random position within the operating volume. In this case, the surface of the sphere possesses three small cubes, which have to be accurately acquired with the appropriate instrument. Once acquisition of a cube has occurred, the application of diathermy is simulated via the depression of a foot pedal. The cube gradually changes colour to reflect the amount of heating applied and vanishes when diathermy has been 'completed'. All three cubes have to be removed. The task is repeated by switching the hands holding the grasping and diathermy instruments.

Task 6: Object manipulation and diathermy

The final task of the original MIST trainer combines the skills acquired in Tasks 4 and 5 and focuses on object acquisition, manipulation and diathermy, within a restrictive volume. An in-theatre example might be accurate instrument replacement of dissecting forceps with a diathermy hook to control precisely a bleeding point on the gall bladder. As before, the system generates a spherical target object at a random position within the operating volume. The subject moves the appropriate instrument tip to acquire the sphere. The remaining instrument is then withdrawn completely from the operating volume. This triggers the system to 'endow' the sphere with a pre-set number of small cubes. The previously withdrawn instrument is then reintroduced into the operating volume and the subject is tasked to apply diathermy to the cubes, only this time the position of the sphere has to be maintained within a small bounding box as well. The task is complete when the set number of cubes have been removed from the sphere. Any unintentional collisions with the sphere and other instrument result in deductions to the accuracy score. The task is repeated by switching the hands holding the grasping and diathermy instruments.

CONCLUSIONS

Subsequent worldwide testing by clinicians and applied psychologists alike have yielded a battery of objective results, one example outcome being that the MIST system now forms a mandatory component of basic and advanced medical courses at the European Surgical Institute near Hamburg, covering a wide range of techniques from cholecystectomy to thoracic surgery. The results include such features as improvements in surgical movement efficiency (actual/ideal instrument path lengths, past-pointing errors and sub-movement corrections) and error reduction when MIST trainees are compared to control groups (eg Taffinder *et al* [27,28,29]). MIST task sensitivity to sleep deprivation has also been shown[30], as have improvements in multiple incision performance, reduction of the Fulcrum Effect (perceived instrument reversal) and increased use of both hands in endoscopic tasks have been reported (Gallagher[31]). In general, it can be stated that experimental results based on MIST tasks demonstrate statistically clear performance differences between novice, junior and experienced laparoscopic cholecystectomy surgeons (Gallagher *et al* [32]).

Of course, MIST is not the only VR-based surgical assessment tool on the market at the present time, although it has been subjected to a more in-depth experimental treatment than many of its contemporaries (approximately five papers delivered during the training session of the September 1999 Annual Scientific Meeting of the Society for Minimally Invasive Therapy were actually based on the MIST system[33]). Companies such as HT Medical are still forging ahead with their own marketable developments. However, MIST is one of the very few systems that has benefited from an initial (if somewhat protracted) human factors analysis. Such an analysis has resulted in a very focused simulation development which not only offers trainers and assessors a structured and validated means of appraising the performance of those in their care, but also allows for future modular expansion, independent of technological developments, in the quest for the comprehensive 'virtual body'. The philosophy underpinning MIST also offers researchers and developers in other domains - operating theatre designers, ergonomics, medical devices and instrument design, for example - a means by which their concepts can be tested by consultant surgeons, thereby minimising the time to market.

As developments in the medical and surgical fields become more and more advanced – in direct intervention/surgery assistance robotics, interactive bespoke patient-imaging techniques and microtechnology, to mention but three – the need for these modular skills simulators will become apparent.

Virtual reality and associated technologies offer enormous potential in the field of early surgical training and in the assessment of perceptual-motor competency/skills at revalidation points of a surgeon's career; this is clear. However, the key to the successful adoption of VR lies not with the hardware and software developers per se, but with a clear user-centred implementation,[34] making sure the technology satisfies the real training and assessment needs of the surgical fraternity of the future.

References

1. Stone RJ. *A Study of the Virtual Reality Market.* UK Department of Trade & Industry. October, 1996.

2. Satava RM. Medicine 2001: The king is dead. In: *Interactive Technology and the New Paradigm for Healthcare.* Washington, DC: IOS Press; 1995. pp334-339.

3. DiGioia AM, Jaramaz B, O'Toole RV, Simon DA, Kanade T. Medical robotics and computer assisted surgery in orthopaedics: An integrated approach. In: *Interactive Technology and the New Paradigm for Healthcare.* Washington, DC: IOS Press; 1995. pp88-90.

4. Adam JA. *Medical electronics.* IEEE Spectrum 1994; 31(1):70-73.

5. Meglan D. Making surgical simulation real. *Computer Graphics* 1996; November: 37-39.

6. http://www.aist.go.jp/NIBH/~b0673/english/cas.html Internet Resources of Computer-aided Surgery by Yasushi Yamauchi.

7. http://www.hitl.washington.edu/projects/knowledge_base/medvr/medvr.html Medicine and Virtual Reality: A Guide to the Literature.Human Interface Technology Laboratory, University of Washington State.

8. Westwood JD, Hoffman HM, Stredney D, Weghorst, SJ, eds. Medicine Meets Virtual Reality 6. *Studies in Health Technology and Informatics,* Volume 50. Washington, DC: IOS Press; 1998.

9. Westwood JD, Hoffman HM, Robb RA, Stredney D, Weghorst, SJ, eds. Medicine Meets Virtual Reality 7. *Studies in Health Technology and Informatics,* Volume 62. Washington, DC: IOS Press; 1999.

10. http://www.nlm.nih.gov/pubs/factsheets/visible_human.html

11. http://iregt1.iai.fzk.de/KISMET/docs/UKMITAT.html

12.   http://robotics.eecs.berkeley.edu/~mdownes/surgery/surgsim.html#Deform

13.   Darzi A, Smith S, Taffinder N. Assessing Operative Skill. *BMJ* 1999; 318:887-888.

14.   http://iac.dtic.mil/cseriac/products/pstoc.html
    The Crew Systems Ergonomics Information Analysis Center is an excellent source of reference material for products and methodologies related to human performance.

15.   Meister D. *Behavior Analysis and Measurement Methods.* New York: Wiley; 1985.

16.   Meister D. *Human Factors Testing and Evaluation.* New York: Elsevier; 1986.

17.   AIAA. *Guide to Human Performance Measurements.* American National Standard (ANSI approved). ANSI/AIAA G-035-1992. 1993.

18.   Endsley MR. Measurement of situation awareness in dynamic systems. *Human Factors* 1995; 37(1):65-84.

19.   Endsley MR. Toward a theory of situation awareness. *Human Factors* 1995; 37(1):32-64.

20.   Bricken W. Training in VR. In: Feldman, T (ed). Virtual Reality '91: Impacts and Applications. *Proceedings of the First Annual Conference on Virtual Reality.* London: Meckler; June 1991.

21.   Terrio FJ, Vreeland JJ. Task Oriented User Requirements and Program Design: an Approach to Writing Programming Objectives and Specifications. *IBM Internal Publication;* August 1980.

22.   Snyder KM. A Guide to Software Usability. *IBM Internal Publication;* 1991.

23.   Stone RJ, McCloy R. Virtual environment training systems for laparoscopic surgery; activities at the UK's Wolfson Centre for Minimally Invasive Therapy. *J Medicine and Virtual Reality* 1996; 1(2):42-51.

24.   Stone RJ. *Interim report: Preliminary findings of an ergonomics study to address working styles and conditions of chicken breast meat and de-boning process operators.* Advanced Robotics Research Ltd. Contract Report (No. ARRL 94.030). March 1994.

25.   Stone RJ. Submersible ergonomics: From theory to practice. In: Megaw ED, ed. *Contemporary Ergonomics. Proceedings of the 1984 Ergonomics Society Conference.* Taylor & Francis; 1984.

26.   Boff KR, Lincoln JE. Engineering Data Compendium: Human Perception and Performance. *Integrated Perceptual Information for Designers Program* (three volumes plus user's guide). HG Armstrong Aerospace Medical Research Laboratory, Wright-Patterson AFB, Ohio; 1988.

27.   Taffinder N, McManus I, Jansen, J, Russell, R, Darzi A. An objective assessment of surgeons' psychomotor skills: Validation of the MISTVR laparoscopic simulator. *B J Surgery* 1998; 85 (Suppl 1):75.

28.   Taffinder N, McManus I, Russell R, Darzi A. An objective assessment of laparoscopic psychomotor skills: the effect of a training course on performance. *Surgical Endoscopy* 1998; 12(5):493.

29.   Taffinder N, Sutton C, Fishwick RJ, McManus IC, Darzi A. Validation of virtual reality to teach and assess psychomotor skills in laparoscopic surgery: Results from randomised controlled studies using the MISTVR laparoscopic simulator. In: Westwood, Hoffman *et al*, eds. *Medicine Meets Virtual Reality.* Washington, DC: IOS Press; 1998. pp124-130.

30.   Taffinder NJ, McManus IC, Gul Y, Russell RCG, Darzi A. Effect of sleep deprivation on surgeons' dexterity on laparoscopy simulator. *The Lancet* 1998; 352:1191.

31.   Gallagher AG, McClure N, McGuigan J, Crothers I, and Browning, J. Virtual reality training in laparoscopic surgery: A preliminary assessment of minimally invasive surgical trainer virtual reality (MISTVR). Presented at: *Medicine Meets Virtual Reality 6*; January 1998; San Diego.

32.   Gallagher AG, Richie K, McClure N, McGuigan J. Psychomotor Skills Assessment of Experienced, Junior and Novice Laparoscopists with Virtual Reality. Internal Note: Northern Ireland Centre for Endoscopic Training and Research. 1999.

33.   Meglan D. Personal communication. 18 September, 1999.

34.   British Standards Institution. ISO 13407. *Human Centred Design Processes for Interactive Systems.* London; 1999.

Assessment of Professional, Clinical and Surgical Skills in the Workplace

CSB Galasko MB, ChM, FRCS(Eng), FRCS(Ed), MSc(Hon)

Professor of Orthopaedic Surgery, University of Manchester

Abstract

A consultant surgeon in the National Health Service requires multiple competencies that are assessed in different ways. Individual assessments of these competencies do not necessarily indicate a surgeon's ability to integrate the different skills required; nor do they assess his/her decision-making ability or judgement, although the latter is probably the most important of all surgical competencies.

The assessment of professional, clinical and surgical skills in the workplace provides a more appropriate means for the assessment of the communication, clinical and surgical skills, as well as the attitude of the trainee surgeon; it is also probably the best way to assess the surgeon's judgement and ability to make decisions.

It is proposed that trainees undergo workplace assessment at three stages in their training — halfway through the training in the generality of their surgical specialty, at the end of training in the generality of their specialty before taking the Intercollegiate Fellowship examination, and at the end of training, when they have completed training both in the generality of their specialty and the advanced sub-specialty training (sub-specialties) of their choice. It is also proposed that training programs should be competence-based rather than based on a specified number of years.

The assessors must be well-trained and the workplace assessment must be objective and reliable. Workplace assessment will be costly to implement but is probably the best way of assessing a surgeon's overall competence.

INTRODUCTION

The full complexities of surgical training and the skills required to be a surgeon are poorly understood; the ability to carry out an operation is only a small, although extremely important, part of the job of a surgeon.

Surgical skills are often compared with those required of an airline pilot. However, if a pilot were to undertake all the roles of the surgeon, he/she would have to interview separately every potential passenger for every flight that he/she was responsible for.

He/she would have to discuss with each passenger where they wanted to go and determine that their destination was the correct one for them (making a diagnosis). He/she would need to determine for each passenger the optimum way of reaching their destination: it may well be that rail, road or sea travel would be better for a particular individual than air travel (advice regarding treatment).

He/she would need to obtain informed consent from every passenger to ensure that they understand what flying involved, including the risks of infection in aircraft, the risks related to the type of ventilation being used for that particular flight, the risks of deep vein thrombosis and pulmonary embolism, the risks of a major air disaster, etc (informed consent).

He/she would need to ensure that every passenger was suitably seated and make alternative arrangements if a flight was overbooked for the onward travel of any passenger who was 'bumped' (organisation of the operating list).

He/she would need to fly the aircraft skilfully from the point of departure to the destination, with the co-pilot and the other crew (carrying out the operation with the surgical, anaesthetic and nursing teams).

Once the aircraft had arrived at its destination, he/she would need to ensure that every passenger was properly looked after and that their journey through Immigration and Customs was free from unnecessary difficulties (immediate post-operative care).

He/she would need to ensure that every passenger reached their ultimate destination safely and that their destination was the correct one for them. He/she would also need to ensure that all the arrangements were in place for them to return home again (post-operative and out-patient care).

And this is only part of a surgeon's job.

Any operation needs to be carried out skilfully. This is the part of a surgeon's job which is comparable to the training of a pilot. The use of a simulator, as used by pilots for each type of plane they fly, is only applicable to a single group of operations for the surgeon. For example, simulation of arthroscopic knee surgery, including the different types of procedures that may be necessary, the complications that may arise and their prevention or management, would be similar to simulation of piloting a 747. It would give no indication of the surgeon's ability to carry out a cruciate ligament reconstruction, an osteotomy around the knee, a total knee replacement, the fixation of a fracture of the upper tibia, the fixation of a fracture of the distal femur, the fixation of a patellar fracture, the management of recurrent dislocation of the patella, nor an operation at any other site in the body. If a surgeon's skill were to be assessed by simulators, dozens of simulators would have to be used for each surgeon, as opposed to one for each plane.

Simulators may, however, be helpful in assessing overall dexterity, rather than an individual surgical procedure or groups of procedures. The use of simulators has been described elsewhere in this book.

Some aspects of technical skills can be assessed by simulators or objective structured assessment of technical skills (OSATS). For example, Martin *et al*[1] described six 15-minute stations which are used to assess tasks such as hand suturing an anastomosis and a stapled anastomosis. These tests assess only a technical skill without saying anything about the operator's understanding of the activity. They cannot be used to assess professional judgement.

It is possible to break down the competencies required to be a competent surgeon and all are necessary for a Certificate of Speciality Training (CCST) in surgery. Each of the following includes a number of sub-sections.

■ Communication, which includes patient counselling, informed consent, imparting bad news such as a terminal illness, communication with other members of the surgical team, and communication with other hospital staff.
■ Knowledge of basic sciences.
■ Knowledge of clinical sciences.
■ Clinical ability (which includes history taking, clinical examination, interpretation of physical symptoms and signs, ability to request relevant investigations, interpret their results and make a diagnosis).

- Decision making and judgement (including a knowledge of the different treatment options, their pros and cons, their likely results and complications, taking into account the individual circumstances of each patient and presenting the treatment options to the patient in a way which the patient can understand).
- Surgical skills and manual dexterity.
- Post-operative management (both in-patient and out-patient).
- Teaching (This includes competencies in teaching, training, appraisal and assessment. All consultants should have the necessary skills to be a trainer, tutor or educational adviser.)
- Learning skills (including self-education).
- Personal effectiveness (including time-management, team-working, team leadership, ethical approach, recognition of ethical dilemmas, attitude, self-criticism, reliability). Reflective behaviour maintains self-criticism and development. There is evidence that this cannot be assumed to be present in all consultants[2] and therefore needs to be taught and assessed at the trainee stage.
- The ability to critically analyse data and interpret the results, interpret both written articles and oral presentations, including audit experience.
- Management skills.

Definitions

The following definitions are used in this article:

Competent – fit for purpose. In this context it means an individual who has all the abilities required to undertake the duties of a consultant surgeon in the National Health Service to an agreed, acceptable standard. It is a standard to be achieved before the issue of a CCST and entry onto the Specialist Register. The *Concise Oxford Dictionary* defines competent as 'adequately qualified'. The division of each competency into knowledge, skills and attitudes is not enough. What is required is the ability to integrate different competencies. It is this integration that is important in judgement and decision-making and the totality of the different competencies required that makes a trained surgeon.

Competencies – this describes the series of abilities that together make up a competent person. It is defined by the *Concise Oxford Dictionary* as 'ability (to do a task)'.

Skill – this is defined by the *Concise Oxford Dictionary* as 'expertness, practised ability, facility (in doing something)'.

Knowledge – there are two components, the general or background body of knowledge that all doctors should possess, plus a more specialised body of knowledge relating to their specific specialty and sub-specialty.

Attitudes – the behaviour of doctors must be compatible with their expected role. It includes the recognition that healthcare is provided within an organisation and not in isolation. It covers ethical behaviour within the UK healthcare setting and clinical governance.

Assessment – in this context, assessment is a summative process that collects evidence about the trainee's progress towards a defined goal and involves making a judgement about whether this goal has been achieved. It is primarily a regulatory process and determines when trainees can move from one stage of training to the next and whether they have reached an appropriate standard for certification. It involves a summative approach to determine whether or not particular competencies have been achieved.

Although the assessment is a summative procedure, it can also be used as a form of appraisal in that areas of weakness can be fed back to the trainee and the trainer so that attention can be given to overcoming these weaknesses. What is important is the overall competence of the individual which will allow him/her to practice as a consultant surgeon within the National Health Service.

Appraisal – is a confidential planned review of progress, focussing on achievements and future activity. It allows training needs to be identified and is primarily concerned with development.

ASSESSMENT

Each of the aforementioned competencies can be separately assessed via a variety of assessments but the most important is the ability to make decisions based on the knowledge gained from using a combination of the above competencies, to judge what is best for a particular patient in particular circumstances, and to be able to inform the patient about their options in a manner that is understood by the patient. A surgeon may have to make 10 – 20 decisions about an individual patient before that patient ever comes to an operating theatre, and possibly just as many in the post-operative period. Although the education required to reach this ability to make decisions has not been quantified, it probably equates, at least, to an MBA.

The question arises as to how best to assess a surgeon's decision-making ability and judgement, particularly as regards patient care. This can be partly assessed by a theoretical examination paper, for example using extended matching questions, but is best tested in a clinical situation. A clinical examination may test the ability to take a history, examine a patient and interpret the findings, but it is an artificial environment. The examinee may feel that further investigations are warranted which may or may not be available to him at the time of the examination. Furthermore, the patient often already knows what treatment has been determined.

It is better, therefore, to assess the skills required to make such decisions in the workplace. Cox[3,4] argued for assessment of performance in practice rather than structured clinical assessments. It is here where surgeons and trainees have to make many decisions every day, in the out-patient clinic, on the ward and in the operating theatre.

Assessment in the workplace

There are two ways in which these skills can be assessed. First, they can be assessed by the trainer with whom the trainee is working. The advantage is that the trainee spends some months working with each trainer. During this period there should be regular appraisals, the trainee's strengths and weaknesses identified, and efforts made to strengthen his 'weak' areas. During this period the trainer should gain an appreciation of the trainee's abilities and be in a position to assess the trainee. The main disadvantage is that the assessment is subjective, although the trainer has the experience of past trainees with which to compare a current trainee. This is the basis of the current United Kingdom higher surgical training program.

Higher surgical training in the United Kingdom is based on a specified number of years as a surgical specialist registrar — six years in most surgical specialties, five years in urology, and oral and maxillofacial surgery. At the end of each post on the training program, trainers are asked to complete an assessment form for each trainee (See Appendix 1). In addition, there exists an annual review process (the RITA – Record of In-Training Assessment process). The review usually involves an interview with an appraisal team which includes the local head of training, representatives of the local training committee, the postgraduate dean or his/her representative and a representative of the local academic department. The appraisal team takes into consideration the assessment forms, the trainee's operating logbook, his/her curriculum vitae and normally an interview with the trainee.

There is, however, a lack of uniformity amongst in-training assessments in different regions. It is for this reason that, ideally, the liaison member from the national Specialist Advisory Committee in that surgical specialty, who is external to the deanery, should be a member of the RITA assessment committee. As indicated above, the RITA process does not objectively assess all the skills required to be a surgeon and there is the possibility that trainees in one deanery may obtain their CCST and entry into the Specialist Register with a lower standard of training than specialist registrars in another region.

At the end of the appraisal one of three forms is issued:
■ record of satisfactory progress within the specialist registrar grade;
■ recommendation for targeted training; or
■ recommendation for intensified supervision/repeated experience or if the trainee has failed to progress following intensified supervision/repeated experience, a recommendation that they be withdrawn from the program.

There are several misconceptions and difficulties with this system. It assumes that all trainees develop at the same rate and, in particular, obtain manual skills at the same rate. Anyone who is slower is deemed to be 'a failure', ie someone who requires remedial action. Training and education at this level should take into account the fact that different individuals acquire different competencies at different rates and, as shown above, a surgeon requires a large number of different competencies. The fact that an individual is acquiring these competencies, albeit more slowly than the average trainee, should not necessarily indicate that he/she requires remedial action. A fixed number of training years also does not take into account the occasional 'high flyer' who obtains these competencies more rapidly than the vast majority of his/her peers.

More importantly, the appraisal scheme as outlined above has its failings. In some instances trainees who are inadequate are not picked up until they have completed several years of training, whereas they should have been counselled at the end of their first or second year that they are not suited for a career in surgery.

The other part of the training program is the specialty examination (the Intercollegiate FRCS). This is taken after the individual has satisfactorily completed four years of training (three years in urology). The individual cannot sit the examination until he/she has obtained a satisfactory fourth year assessment. Nevertheless, 15 to 20% of trainees fail the examination, indicating that they have not reached the competencies required for someone in his/her fifth year of training (fourth year in urology), even though the RITA process has suggested that they have.

The examination is an excellent way of assessing knowledge and can be used to assess the ability to take a history and examine a patient. It does not assess surgical or manual dexterity skills and, as indicated above, is not ideal for assessing the ability to make decisions and exercise judgement. It can be used to assess communication skills and the ability to critically analyse data.

Secondly, objective assessments can be undertaken by trained external observers. This overcomes many of the above difficulties. It is essential that the assessment is objective, that the assessors are external, that they assess a number of trainees each year and that the assessment is carried out in the workplace. If it is, the trainee can be assessed carrying out some of the more important skills required to be a surgeon.

The assessors would spend one or two days observing the trainee conducting an out-patient clinic, seeing both old and new patients, examining them, requesting and interpreting the results of investigations, making diagnoses, advising patients and their families about treatment, counselling patients and obtaining from them informed consent. During the visit some time would be spent on a ward round where the trainee will be assessed seeing patients both pre-operatively and post-operatively, sorting out any pre-operative problems, counselling patients, obtaining informed consent, ensuring that their post-operative progress is smooth, dealing with complications, and maintaining adequate pain relief. Finally, the trainee would carry out an operating list, probably assisted by the trainer, the procedures carried out being selected from those which, according to the logbook, the trainee has been assessed as being competent to do without supervision. Surgical skills and manual dexterity would be assessed, as well as the ability to cope with any unexpected findings such as anatomical variations. Not only would this give an assessment of the trainee's decision-making and judgement skills, clinical skills, surgical skills and manual dexterity, but would also assess communication and personal effectiveness skills.

No single method is sufficient to provide an adequate assessment of the competence of a trainee. A true picture only comes from a variety of assessment tools but assessment in the workplace is essential.

The Standing Committee on Postgraduate Medical and Dental Education (SCOPME) has emphasised the need to look at performance in the workplace. SCOPME also embraced the concept that Limen referencing (which relates the standard of the trainee's performance to that of an assessor's expert understanding of the minimum for safe practice) could provide the basis for a workplace assessment standard.[5] Such an approach has been found to be useful and reliable amongst anaesthetists in

Australia.[6] Although it may be difficult to quantify the element of professional judgement involved, there is currently no better single published test of assessing performance of the whole task.[7] Inherently included in the assessment are the trainee's qualities of judgement, team-working and professionalism in their widest context.

The Royal College of Anaesthetists has already established a pilot scheme in South Thames (East) in which trainees are observed working on a routine operating list by an external assessor. The trainee's overall approach to pre-operative assessment, communication with the patient, anaesthetic procedures and post-operative care is assessed against recognised standards of clinical practice.[8] The results of this and other assessments were a major influence in the College wanting to extend their specialist registrar training program by one year.

Assessing attitudes, judgement and professionalism are the most difficult, the most subjective and yet ultimately perhaps the most important parts of the program of training. Aspects of personality and life style (for example unavailability at short notice when on call, persistent lateness wasting operating theatre time, attitudes that recurrently produce conflict in the working environment) are just as important to patient care as the ability to understand key aspects of pharmacology or monitoring.[8]

The Medical Protection Society[9] has recently reviewed 337 surgical claims across a range of surgical specialties. The causes of the claim were classified as follows:

Intra-operative problems	34%
Failure to recognise complication	19%
Failure to make post-operative observations	7%
Delay in performing procedure	7%
Failing to warn/consent issues	6%
Infusion problems, equipment malfunction, diathermy burns and improper delegation	5%
Operation not indicated	5%
Wrong diagnosis	5%
Unexpected death	4%
Failure to interpret radiographs	3%
Wrong part operated upon	3%
Foreign body left *in situ*	2%

Most of these problems would not be assessed in a formal examination, but would be in the workplace.

The clinical material reviewed contained a huge variation in the type of procedures undertaken for a range of very differing diagnoses. However, the areas of concern related to more general aspects of care which could occur in any specialty and which were potentially avoidable were:

■ misinterpretation of histological specimens and results leading to unnecessary or inappropriate procedures;

■ problems with technique in minimally invasive surgery;

■ unrecognised organ damage in open procedures and subsequent delay in recognising post-operative deterioration;

■ delay in undertaking surgery due to failure to recognise need;

■ operative procedure not indicated, because of communication failure, surgeon's inexperience or error of clinical judgement;

■ failure to warn in cases where patients have not been informed of relevant and significant risks which would have affected their decision making; and

■ initial incorrect diagnoses leading to the performance of inappropriate procedures with inadequate consent.

It must be emphasised that the assessors need to be trained so that they are able to objectively and accurately assess the trainee's skills[10] and, as with all methods of assessment,[11] workplace assessment must be shown to be reliable.

Cost

The question arises as to how often these assessments should be carried out. They will be expensive, particularly with respect to surgeons' time. Highly skilled, trained surgeons will be required to undertake these assessments, necessitating them to be away from their workplace. Ways will have to be found to ensure that the work continues to be done in their Trust.

For assessments to be fair and to be seen to be fair, they must be undertaken by more than one person. It is important, therefore, that two visitors carry out the workplace assessment.

As no surgeon will undertake an assessment role on a full-time basis (he/she will still need to continue with their own clinical practice) and assuming that two assessors will carry out each assessment and each trainee will be assessed, on average, every two years, the additional number of surgeons that will need to be appointed to cover this work will be between 30 and 40. This will be the main cost of this form of assessment. The appointment of these additional surgeons will not increase the number of patients treated, but will allow assessors to spend some weeks each year carrying out this duty. In addition to the salaries of the extra consultants, there will be the cost of travel, overnight accommodation, and secretarial and administrative staff to organise the visits and administer the reports.

Gonczi[12] and Hager[13] have also described an 'integrated' model of competence assessment that has been adopted by a number of professions in Australia and have also acknowledged that this system is expensive to deliver.

Training and appointment of assessors

The assessors will need to be trained and should be chosen on merit, having demonstrated above average knowledge of the subject as well as proven skills in assessing. The assessors should be chosen by open competition. There should be a clear job description laying out the requirements of the position and explaining that they will be required to attend a course. They should be prepared to give up a minimum of two to three weeks a year, as do MRCS examiners. They should probably serve for a minimum of six years, three years as the junior member of an assessment team and three years as the senior.

The training course will include an evaluation of an assessor's ability to carry out the assessment reliably and competently. It must show how the behaviour of the visitor is crucial in providing a fair assessment of the trainee. They need to be able to manage dysfunctional trainees and provide comprehensive and clear reports as to why a trainee has or has not successfully completed the assessment. They must provide an assessment that can be seen to be robust, consistent, capable of validation, accountable and comprehensive.

In the assessment of real-world consultations, no two trainees see the same patients. It is impossible, therefore, to pre-set specific criteria for the assessment of the consultation. Reliance must be placed upon the experience and expertise of the examiner and his or her ability to recognise competent practice in new situations (Limen referencing).

The assessors will need to develop the internal construct of competence which takes cognisance of the components. Criteria will need to be identified before the assessment takes place and different assessors will need to stick to the same categories of competence.

Establishing criteria for assessment

One asks 'what is to be measured?' It is not possible to measure competence until one is clear what specialist registrars should be able to do. It is necessary to:

■ define the knowledge, skills and attitudes to be exhibited and measured;

■ define what standard of performance is required; and

■ define under what conditions the assessment will be made.

Frequency of assessments

Higher surgical training occurs in two stages:

■ training in the generality of the specialty (for example general surgery, trauma and orthopaedic surgery, neurosurgery); and

■ training in an advanced sub-specialty (sub-specialties) within the main surgical specialty. For example, in general surgery it may include breast surgery, vascular surgery, colo-proctology, etc, whereas in orthopaedic surgery it may include spinal surgery, upper limb surgery, knee surgery, children's orthopaedic surgery, etc.

It is proposed that an external assessment be carried out at three stages in surgical training:

■ halfway through training in the generality of the specialty. This is roughly equivalent to an average trainee at the end of two years of specialist registrar training;

■ at the end of training in the generality of the specialty. This is roughly equivalent to the average trainee at the end of his/her fourth year of training; and

■ at the end of training. This assessment would be in the generality of the specialty, as well as the trainee's chosen sub-specialty (sub-specialties) in which they have received advanced surgical training. This would be at the end of surgical training, at the time that they would be recommended for a CCST and for entry onto the Specialist Register.

The development of such a program will identify a range of competencies which a surgeon should achieve at different levels in training, including the competencies required for entry onto the Specialist Register. It will also establish the level of skill in each competency required at different levels of training.

Because the assessment will be carried out by external, trained assessors, it should be defensible and able to withstand challenge from surgeons-in-training who have not achieved the required level.

The workplace assessment will need to evaluate the breadth of clinical experience and not just the number of operations undertaken or procedures observed.

Before such assessments can be established or even pilot studies examined, the national Specialist Advisory Committee in each surgical specialty will have to define the level of skill in each of the competencies required by a trainee halfway through their training in the generality of their specialty; at the end of training in the generality of surgery before they embark upon advanced surgical training; and at the end of training, both in the generality of the surgical specialty and in each sub-specialty. On successful completion of the assessments, trainees will be recommended for a CCST and entry onto the Specialist Register.

No operation is always successful. Every procedure has its complications and failures. These are often given as a percentage average when risks are discussed with the patient and/or the family. Poloniecki[14] has pointed out that half of the surgeons will be below the average results and one will have the worst result. It is essential, therefore, that all surgeons gain the minimal level of competence required for consultant surgical practice in the NHS. In order to achieve this, the skills required in all the competencies needed to be a competent surgeon have to be defined and assessed. Klein[15] concluded that there may be a need for more explicit and stringent training requirements before surgeons are permitted to operate independently. Currently, there is no external assessment of surgical skills and it is left to the trainers using the assessment forms shown in Appendix 1. The clinical evaluation on site will provide this external and objective assessment. When the trainee and his/her trainers feel that the trainee has reached the necessary level of expertise for that stage of training, a clinical evaluation on site will be requested.

Some trainees have requested that their CCST date be deferred as they did not feel confident enough to take on independent practice. This is a major drawback with a training program based on a specified number of years. In surgery, operative totals should not be used. It is more important that the surgeon can carry out an operation competently, have the professional judgement to know when an operation is indicated and is able to care for the patient post-operatively, than to just count numbers of operations undertaken. Some individuals are naturally gifted technical surgeons, whereas others require much more training to develop the same level of manual dexterity and operative expertise. External assessment in the workplace will give a better objective view of a surgeon's technical ability than just counting the number of operations, as indicated in the logbook. Nevertheless, a minimum number of procedures must be carried out for the trainee to obtain the experience necessary to deal with the unexpected.

If this system is adopted, there will be several advantages. First, it will lay down the competencies required at different stages of training, based on stages rather than years of training. When a trainee and his/her trainers believe that the trainee has reached the level of competence required for that stage of training, an external assessment will be sought. Some trainees may reach the level required for their first assessment after 18 months, others may require 30 months, but those that take longer will not be regarded as 'failures' who require remedial action once training becomes competency based, rather than based on the specific duration of training.

If a trainee does not reach the level of skills required, he/she will need to be counselled. This will be particularly important at the first assessment when a decision will need to be made whether the trainee should be removed from the training program or counselled as to where their weaknesses are and how to correct them. In the latter instance, a further assessment will be required after six months' further training. Once they have satisfactorily reached the level of skills required at the first stage, the second part of their training can commence.

At the second stage, the assessment will be used to help determine whether the trainee is adequately skilled in the generality of his specialty to allow him to undertake advanced training in the sub-specialty of his choice, or whether he/she requires further training because their personal judgement, such as clinical skills and/or surgical skills, have not yet developed to the extent where they can be considered to have reached the competencies required for the completion of training in the generality of their specialty. Once they have reached the second level of skill, they will be able to sit the specialty examination and if they pass that, will be able to embark upon advanced surgical training.

Once they have reached the third level of skill, they will be competent to be entered onto the Specialist Register and practise as a consultant surgeon within the NHS. When someone has reached this level of competence, he/she will need to continue with their self-education and professional development for the rest of their careers. Part of the assessment must be to ensure that they are able to do so.

The results of the workplace assessment will have to be fed back to the trainee and trainer and cannot be considered in isolation. They must be considered together with the other assessments used to determine the level of competence reached by the trainee in the other skills required to become a surgeon.

The workplace assessment should also be helpful in determining where there are weaknesses and, as such, should be used as part of appraisal as well as the assessment.

Competency-based assessment

The Specialist Training Authority of the Royal Medical Colleges is bound by the minimum periods of training specified in European legislation. It may, therefore, never be possible to move entirely away from a minimum period of training, but most surgical training in the United Kingdom takes longer than that specified in European legislation. The development of a competency-based assessment may reduce the duration of training for a high flyer, who is a naturally gifted technical surgeon, but it is unlikely that the reduction in the time taken to reach the competencies required to become a consultant will be less than that required by European legislation.

Although assessment in the workplace has profound disadvantages in terms of cost and logistics and has not yet been shown to be reproducible, it is the best method currently available for assessing training posts and as such, is relied upon by the Hospital Recognition Committee of The Royal College of Surgeons of England as the mainstay for the supervision of basic surgical training and by the Joint Committee on Higher Surgical Training of the United Kingdom and Ireland via its Specialist Advisory Committee in each surgical specialty, for the supervision of higher surgical training in the different surgical specialties. Therefore, there exists a precedent for such visits. It cannot, however, replace the current Intercollegiate Specialty examination, but serves to complement it. It also serves to complement the assessments of the other competencies required to make a competent surgeon, as described above.

It must be emphasised that the assessment of professional, clinical and surgical skills in the workplace will not assess every skill required to be a surgeon. Other assessments will also be required. The trainee will need to continue to have regular appraisals and assessments from their trainers: for example, they will need to be tested on their knowledge base. The advantages of this system over the current system are that it will be objective, will define more accurately all the competencies required to be a surgeon and in particular the clinical, surgical and judgement/decision-making skills, it will be able to assess them more accurately and more objectively than current methods of assessment, and will make training competency rather than time-based.

The Specialist Training Authority of the Medical Royal Colleges, which is the statutory body that recommends individuals to have their names entered on the Specialist Register, requires a clear definition of the competencies required by individual trainees for the award of CCST. The development of a workplace assessment scheme, as described above, will achieve this, particularly with respect to the clinical and operative competencies required to be a consultant surgeon.

Probably the most difficult competency to assess, but also the most important, is professional judgement. It is suggested that this scheme, if properly funded and instituted, should be able to assess this competency. It will enable problems in early training to be identified. It will identify for program directors, trainers and trainees what competencies are required at different stages of training. It will create more standardisation and objectivity in assessment throughout the United Kingdom.

Both the New Deal[16] and the Calman Training Programme[17] have resulted in a significant reduction in the time available to train a surgeon and, therefore, it is essential to define the competencies required for an individual to be competent to practise as a consultant surgeon in the NHS, particularly at a time when the surgeon's capabilities are being more critically analysed by patients and government. It is suggested that the above scheme of defining the competencies required, the level of skill needed in each competency at different levels of training, the use of a number of assessments, and the assessment of professional, clinical and surgical skills in the workplace will provide confidence to trainees, patients and government that surgical trainees are competent to work as a consultant surgeon in the NHS once they have satisfactorily completed training and obtained their CCST.

If this proves successful, a similar external assessment in the workplace could become part of the mechanism of the quinquennial revalidation of consultant surgeons.

References

1.   Martin G, Regehr R, Reznick H, MacRae J Murnaghan J. Objective structured assessment of technical skills (OSTS) for surgical residents. *B J Surg* 1997; 87:273-278.

2.   Klemola U-M, Norros L. Analysis of the clinical behaviour of anaesthetists; recognition of uncertainty as a basis for practice. *Medical Education* 1997; 31:449-456.

3.   Cox K. No Oscar for OSCA. *Medical Education* 1990; 24:540-545.

4.   Cox K. What surgeons know. A note on clinical working knowledge. *Aus NZ J Surg* 1992; 62:836-840.

5.   SCOPME. *Appraising Doctors and Dentists in Training. Working Paper for Consultation.* London; 1996. pp26-27.

6.   Paget NS, Newble DI, Saunders NA, Du J. Physician assessment pilot study for the Royal Australasian College of Physicians. *J Continuing Educ in the Health Professions* 1996; 16:103-111.

7.   Jolly B, Grant J. *The Good Assessment Guide.* London: Joint Centre for Education in Medicine; 1997.

8.   Royal College of Anaesthetists. *Assessment of Trainees.* London; 1998.

9.   Medical Protection Society. Can the society help me avoid the possible pitfalls of practice? *Strength (The Medical Protection Society Review)* 1998; 6-7.

10.   Jolly B, Wakeford R, Newble D. Requirements for action and research in certification and recertification. In: Newble D, Jolly B, Wakeford R, eds. *The Certification and Recertification of Doctors: Issues in the Assessment of Clinical Competence.* Cambridge: Cambridge University Press; 1994. pp231-249.

11.   Van der Vletuen C, Newble D. Methods of assessment in certification. In: Newble D, Jolly B, Wakeford R, eds. *The Certification and Recertification of Doctors: Issues in the Assessment of Clinical Competence.* Cambridge: Cambridge University Press; 1994. pp105-125.

12.   Gonczi A. Competency based assessment in the professions in Australia. *Assessment in Education* 1994; 1:27-44.

13.   Hager P, Gonczi A. What is competence? *Medical Teacher* 1996; 18:15-18.

14.   Poloniecki J. Half of all doctors are below average. *BMJ* 1998; 316:1734-1736.

15.   Klein R. Competence, professional self regulation and the public interest. *BMJ* 1998; 316:1740-1742.

16.   National Health Service Medical Executive. *The New Deal: Plan for Action.* The Report of the Working Group on Specialist Medical Training. Leeds; 1994.

17.   Department of Health. *Hospital Doctors: Training for the Future.* The Report of the Working Group in Medical Training. Leeds: Department of Health; 1993.

Appendix 1.

JOINT COMMITTEE ON HIGHER SURGICAL TRAINING
TRAINEE ASSESSMENT FORM

This is an official document. The original is the property of the JCHST. For the annual assessment process the JCHST office will make the forms available, on request, to the Programme Directors who will supervise their completion by the appropriate trainer(s). The forms will be signed upon completion, by the trainer(s) and the trainee <u>before</u> the <u>original copy is returned to the JCHST</u> office at the Royal College of Surgeons of England. Photocopies of the forms should be passed to the Programme Director, the Trainer(s), Regional Postgraduate Dean and the Intercollegiate Board if the appropriate <u>only</u>. <u>Please ensure that the details in the box below are completed, this form will be returned if incomplete, resulting in a delay for process.</u>

TRAINEE:	NTN/TN/FTN OR LAT:
SPECIALTY:	YEAR: 6mths 1 2 3 4 5 6
ROTATION:	HOSPITAL:
PERIOD COVERED FROM:	TO:

CRITERIA	POOR	DEFICIENT	SATISFACTORY the majority of trainees	GOOD	EXCELLENT	COMMENTS
A. Clinical Skills						
History taking						
Physical exam						
Investigators						
Diagnosis						
Judgement						
Operative skill						
After care						
B. Knowledge						
Basic science						
Clinical						
C. Post grad activities						
Teaching						
Lecturing style						
Case presentation						
Presentations						
Publications						
Research ability and audit						

CRITERIA	POOR	DEFICIENT	SATISFACTORY the majority of trainees	GOOD	EXCELLENT	COMMENTS
D. Attitude						
Reliability						
Self motivation						
Leadership						
Administration						
Relationships with						
a) colleagues						
b) patients						
c) other staff						

TRAINERS PEN PICTURE:

TRAINERS SIGNATURE(S): _____ / _____ DATE: _____
and NAME in block capitals
_____ / _____ DATE: _____
_____ / _____ DATE: _____
_____ / _____ DATE: _____
TRAINEE SIGNATURE: _____ / _____ DATE: _____

SIGNATURE OF THE TRAINEE INDICATES THAT HE/SHE HAS SEEN THE ASSESSMENT FORM, NOT THAT HE/SHE AGREES WITH IT'S CONTENT.

Trainees who disagree with the contents of this report may appeal in the first instance to the appropriate Specialist Advisory Committee and thence to the JCHST.

NOTES TO ACCOMPANY JCHST TRAINEE ASSESSMENT FORM

1.   The Assessment Form is CONFIDENTIAL once completed, and must be handled accordingly.

2.   The following guidelines are for trainers completing the form

   a. complete as fully as possible the trainee details in the top box, circling the appropriate year of assessment.

   b. Where more then one trainer is involved with the trainee a consensus opinion should be expressed on the form, which should be signed by all trainers.

   c. Complete the main assessment by placing an 'X' in one box only against each criterion. The comments box is available for additional comment if desired. the following guidelines are to be used when grading criteria. (SACs would expect most trainees to be graded SATISFACTORY if their training is progressing to a standard which would see them being recommended for the CCST).

3.   THE FORM WILL BE RETURNED IF INCOMPLETE.

	POOR/DEFICIENT	SATISFACTORY	GOOD/EXCELLENT
A. Clinical Skills			
History taking	Incomplete. Inaccurate. Poorly recorded	Usually complete, orderly and systematic	Precise, perceptive, 'can spot the rarity'
Physical exam	Lacks basic skill. Relies unnecessarily on investigations.	Can elicit correct signs. Recognises most significant findings.	Thorough, accurate. Knows and elicits specialist signs
Diagnosis	Fails to interpret and synthesise symptoms, and investigations.	Competent clinician. Good knowledge with an orderly logical approach to differential diagnosis.	Outstanding diagnostician. Excellent clinical memory
Judgement	Unreliable. Fails to grasp significance of findings or take appropriate action. Under or over reacts to emergencies	Reliable. Competent under pressure. Asks for advice appropriately.	Outstanding clinician who is aware of his/her limits.
Operative skill	Clumsy, rough with tissues. Totally lacking in self confidence technically.	Competent. Handles tissues well. Reliable endoscopist.	A master technician, in both open and endoscopic surgery.
After care	Uninterested. Fails to notice complications and act appropriately.	Conscientious. Good awareness for complications Reliable in outpatients.	Excellent on wards. Notices problems early. Outstanding in follow up outpatients.

	POOR/DEFICIENT	SATISFACTORY	GOOD/EXCELLENT
B. Knowledge			
History taking	Uninterested, does not read literature. Fails to apply basic science to clinical problems.	Adequate fund knowledge and relates this satisfactorily to patient care.	Outstanding knowledge and understanding of the basic science of the speciality. Widely read.
Clinical	Poorly read. Lacks appropriate knowledge to construct a differential diagnosis. Fails to learn from experience.	Satisfactory knowledge for dealing with the common disorders. May fail to 'spot the rarity' but learns from experience.	Outstanding knowledge. Can be relied upon to 'spot the rarity'. Widely read.

	POOR/DEFICIENT	SATISFACTORY	GOOD/EXCELLENT
C. Postgraduate Activities			
Teaching	Uninterested and avoids teaching Contributes little to the education of students or trainees in the grades below e.g. SHOs.	Competent and conscientious in teaching others	Excellent enthusiastic teacher. Can inspire.
Lecturing style	Avoids if possible. Poor style, poorly delivered, boring.	Reasonably well delivered. Competent but lacking spark.	Excellently delivered. Dynamic. Logical and clear Can 'hold' audience
Case presentation	Poor on history, signs diagnosis and discussion.	Competent. History and signs correct. Good deductions.	Excellent presentation and discussion.
Presentations	No interest in giving papers When has to, does it badly. Fails to get message across.	Keen to give presentations which are well illustrated and well delivered.	Fully researched. Original ideas. Answers questions lucidly.
Publications	Shows no interest. Devoid of ideas. No grasp of English.	Keen, tries hard but lacking originality. Reasonable grasp of English.	An excellent CV. Many original ideas which are translated into published articles.
Research ability and audit	Has neither the inclination or ideas. Unable to carry out 'directed' projects. Not interested in audit.	Keen to do research and/or audit but need considerable direction. Reasonable grasp of statistics and research methods	Flair for original research with ability to carry out independently. Utilises effective research methods.

	POOR/DEFICIENT	SATISFACTORY	GOOD/EXCELLENT
D. Attitudes			
Reliability	Unreliable, scatterbrained. Forgets to do things to the possible detriment of patients	Dependable. Does not need reminding. Conscientious in patient care.	Highly conscientious. Anticipates problems.
Self motivation	No inclination to organise work. Needs to be 'pushed' constantly.	Able to organise working routine without supervision. Looks for opportunities to learn.	Constantly pro-active, always prepared to accept additional opportunities to advance.
Leadership	Very limited. 'Switches people off'. Colleagues and other staff confused by his/her instructions.	Competent but lacks inspiration. Gives clear instructions.	Outstanding team leader with exceptional ability to inspire others.
Administration	Can not be bothered. Always behind with letters and summaries. 'In a permanent muddle'.	Conscientious. Can be confidently left to deal with letters, summaries, waiting lists etc.	Excellent at routine administration. Has a good grasp of hospital management and politics.

	POOR/DEFICIENT	SATISFACTORY	GOOD/EXCELLENT
E. Relationships with:			
a. Colleagues	Fails to get on with seniors, contemporaries or juniors. May even undermine them.	Good rapport with colleagues Usually willing to help in a crisis. Trusted, easy to work with.	Always willing to help even if personally inconvenient. Able to defuse problems in the surgical team. 'An excellent colleague'.
b. Patients	Increases patients anxieties. Rude. Patient do not want him/her as their doctor. Bad listener and communicator.	Sound caring attitude. Can allay patients fears. Takes time. Listens well, explains well. Trusted by patient.	Inspires confidence. Establishes good rapport. Excellent communicator. Patients delighted to be looked after by him/her.
c. Other staff	Treats them with disdain. Generates as opposed to solving problems.	Sound and professional yet approachable. Treats others with respect and is respected in turn.	Inspires enthusiasm. Exceptional communication skills.

Pen picture

Please summarise the trainee's character and overall performance drawing attention to any outstanding features or alternatively ways which the the trainee failed to to meet your expectations during this rotation. Do you foresee any specific difficulties/gaps in training that the trainee will have in completing his/her training?